T0281573

Rapid Reference Review in Sports Medicine

Pivotal Papers Revealed

Editors

Mark D. Miller, MD
S. Ward Casscells Professor of Orthopaedic Surgery
University of Virginia
Charlottesville, Virginia
Team Physician
James Madison University
Harrisonburg, Virginia

Cyril Mauffrey, MD, FACS, FRCS
Director of Orthopaedic Trauma
Denver Health Medical Center
Associate Professor of Orthopaedic Surgery
University of Colorado School of Medicine
Aurora, Colorado

David J. Hak, MD, MBA, FACS
Professor
Orthopedic Surgery, University of Colorado
Denver Health Medical Center
Denver, Colorado

Contributing Editors

Megan M. Gleason, MD
Resident Physician
Department of Orthopaedic Surgery
University of Virginia
Charlottesville, Virginia

Jeff Tuman, MD
Slocum Center for Orthopedics and Sports
Medicine
Eugene, Oregon

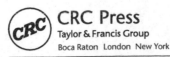

CRC Press
Taylor & Francis Group
Boca Raton London New York

CRC Press is an imprint of the
Taylor & Francis Group, an **informa** business

First published 2016 by SLACK Incorporated

Published 2024 by CRC Press
2385 NW Executive Center Drive, Suite 320, Boca Raton FL 33431

and by CRC Press
4 Park Square, Milton Park, Abingdon, Oxon, OX14 4RN

CRC Press is an imprint of Taylor & Francis Group, LLC

© 2016 Taylor & Francis Group, LLC

Visit the Taylor & Francis Web site at
http://www.taylorandfrancis.com

and the CRC Press Web site at
http://www.crcpress.com

Library of Congress Cataloging-in-Publication Data

Miller, Mark D., author.
  Rapid reference review in sports medicine : pivotal papers revealed / Mark D. Miller, Cyril Mauffrey, David J. Hak.
    p. ; cm.
    Includes bibliographical references.
    ISBN 9781617118326 (hardback)
    I. Mauffrey, Cyril, author. II. Hak, David J., author. III. Title.
    [DNLM: 1. Sports Medicine--Abstracts. ZQT 261]
    Z6667.W6
    [RD97]
    016.6171'027--dc23
                              2015023461

ISBN: 9781617118326 (pbk)
ISBN: 9781003526254 (ebk)

DOI: 10.1201/9781003526254

Dedication

To all sports medicine enthusiasts in search of "the classics."
Mark D. Miller, MD

This book is dedicated to my residents and fellows.
Cyril Mauffrey, MD, FACS, FRCS

For Kimberly and Hailey, the pivotal people in my life.
David J. Hak, MD, MBA, FACS

Contents

About the Editors

Mark D. Miller, MD is the Head of the Division of Sports Medicine and the S. Ward Casscells Professor of Orthopaedic Surgery at the University of Virginia. He is a Distinguished Graduate of the Air Force Academy and the Uniformed Services University F. Edward Hebert' School of Medicine. Dr. Miller is a highly decorated retired Colonel in the US Air Force and former team physician for the US Air Force Academy. He currently serves as team physician for James Madison University in Harrisonburg, Virginia. Dr. Miller has over 25 orthopaedic textbooks that he has written and/or edited including the "best selling" Review of Orthopaedics (now in its 7th Edition) and is the author of over 200 peer reviewed articles. He is the Founder/Director of the popular Miller Review Course, and is a highly sought after speaker.

Dr. Miller has been very active in several professional societies including the American Orthopaedic Society for Sports Medicine (AOSSM), and is the former chair for three different committees in that society. He was an American Orthopaedic Association North American Traveling Fellow and both a Traveling Fellow and a Godfather for the AOSSM Traveling Fellowship program. Dr. Miller has been named as a "Top Doctor" for numerous regional, national, and international programs. Although widely known for his expertise in knee surgery, Dr. Miller is also an accomplished shoulder surgeon and sports medicine specialist. He is married to his wife, Ann, and has four grown children and two grandchildren.

Cyril Mauffrey, MD, FACS, FRCS is the director of Orthopaedic Trauma at Denver Health Medical Center. He was trained in the United Kingdom and obtained his Orthopaedic boards through the Royal College of Surgeons. Following a year at the University Hospital of Louisville as an Orthopaedic Trauma fellow, he joined Denver Health Medical Center and the University of Colorado School of Medicine where he is an Associate Professor. Dr. Mauffrey's research and clinical interest include novel strategies for the management of long bone infections in addition to pelvic and acetabular fractures. Dr. Mauffrey is the Editor in Chief for the *European Journal of Orthopaedic Surgery and Traumatology* and on the board of directors of the International Society for Fracture Repair (ISFR) alongside other organizations such as SICOT and the OTA.

David J. Hak, MD, MBA, FACS graduated from the University of Michigan and received his medical degree from Ohio State University. His postdoctoral training included an orthopedic residency at the University of California at Los Angeles and an orthopedic trauma fellowship at the

University of California at Davis. He received his MBA in health care administration from Auburn University. He has been on the faculty of the University of Michigan, the University of California at Davis, and the University of Colorado. Dr. Hak is a fellow of the American Academy of Orthopaedic Surgeons and the American College of Surgeons. He serves in various leadership roles in the Orthopaedic Trauma Association and the International Society for Fracture Repair.

Introduction

Attempting to select "pivotal" papers is undoubtedly a nearly impossible task, which by necessity leaves out hundreds of equally important, or even more important, articles. To achieve a concise list of "pivotal" papers, the following criteria have been considered:

1. Prospective, randomized clinical studies (level I evidence)
2. Large prospective clinical cohort studies
3. Meta-analyses of published series on controversial topics
4. Articles that are commonly cited, either in the literature or during teaching conferences
5. Selections from *Top 100 Cited Articles in Clinical Orthopedic Sports Medicine*
6. When possible, we have focused on clinical studies, rather than anatomic or biomechanical studies

In addition, there is wide variability in the number of potential "pivotal" papers to select from on different topics. Therefore, some chapters may have articles that you may consider of relatively low importance and other chapters may omit well-designed prospective randomized clinical trials. There is also wide variation in the rigor of individual studies, since they span many decades during which research and publication standards have changed.

The exclusion of any article from this text should not lead the reader to minimize its worth. Invariably the authors of these other articles are well justified in feeling slighted and can rightfully question why their article was not included. As already mentioned, any attempt to select "pivotal" articles is an impossible task given the wide range of important and worthwhile papers.

As the medical information expands at an exponential pace, the ability to quickly identify relevant articles using PubMed becomes increasingly difficult. It is our hope that readers will find this text useful in their education and practice. Orthopedic trainees may be able to quickly review several articles in preparation for a morning conference presentation of patients with a specific injury, and practicing surgeons may be able to advise patients on the relative benefits of one treatment over another.

In addition to pivotal papers, we have included selected review articles for many of the chapters. Additional review materials can also be found in the American Academy of Orthopedic Surgeons Instructional Course Lectures and in the Cochrane Reviews.

We are all indebted to the hard work of the authors of articles reviewed in this text, for their efforts and knowledge are what have helped us all advance the care of our patients. Any errors and omissions in the material presented is our responsibility, not that of the original authors.

Finally, although we have attempted to abstract the key findings from each paper, we would encourage you to read the complete paper for a thorough understanding of the methods and findings. Like any review book, these annotated references are intended to serve as a guide and not as a replacement for the original work. The reader may also notice differences in numbers reported in this text with those in the papers' abstracts. Abstracts often refer to the total number of patients eligible for study, and for clarity we have usually tried to provide the numbers used in the final data analysis.

Standard abbreviations/notations used in the text:

- ACL = anterior cruciate ligament
- CT = computed tomography
- DVT = deep vein thrombosis
- LCL = lateral collateral ligament
- MCL = medial collateral ligament
- MPa = megapascal
- MRI = magnetic resonance imaging
- N = Newton
- PCL = posterior cruciate ligament
- preop = preoperative
- post-op = post-operative
- SF = short form
- + = standard deviation
- ° = degrees

Where a set of 2 numbers appears in parentheses, this indicates the associated range of values, for example: Average age 38 years (22 to 68 years).

David J. Hak, MD, MBA, FACS

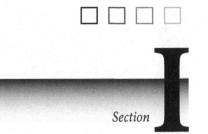

Section

I

Knee

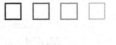

Knee Anatomy, Biomechanics, and Clinical Rating Systems

Chapter **1**

FEATURED ARTICLE

Authors: Butler DL, Boyes FR, Grood ES.

Title: Ligamentous restraints to anterior-posterior drawer in the human knee: a biomechanical study.

Journal Information: *J Bone Joint Surg Am*. 1980;62:259–270.

Study Design: Cadaveric Study

▶ This study ranked the order of importance of each ligament and capsular structure in resisting the clinical anterior and posterior drawer tests.

▶ This study quantified the functions of the ligaments by measuring individual restraining forces during precisely controlled, single-plane, anterior-posterior tibial displacement.

▶ 14 cadaveric knees were studied:

  ▷ 11 tested in 90 degrees of knee flexion

  ▷ 3 tested in 30 degrees of knee flexion

▶ Specimens were mounted in an Instron testing machine, with the femur secured to a load cell and the tibia secured to a moving actuator.

▶ Structures were cut in varying order among specimens:

  ▷ Anterior cruciate ligament (ACL)

  ▷ Posterior cruciate ligament (PCL)

  ▷ Iliotibial tract and band

  ▷ Midmedial capsule

Miller MD, Mauffrey C, Hak DJ.
Rapid Reference Review in Sports Medicine:
Pivotal Papers Revealed (pp 3-25).
© 2016 Taylor & Francis Group.

▷ Midlateral capsule

▷ Medial collateral ligament (MCL)

▷ Lateral collateral ligament (LCL)

▶ The authors introduced the concept of primary and secondary ligament restraints.

Results: Anterior Drawer Constraints

▶ The ACL is the primary restraint to the anterior drawer, providing an average of 86% of the total resisting force.

▶ All other ligaments and capsular structures provide the remaining secondary restraint, each typically contributing < 3% of the total resisting force.

Results: Posterior Drawer Constraints

▶ The PCL is the primary restraint to the posterior drawer.

▶ The posterior lateral capsule, popliteus tendon, and the MCL provided the greatest secondary restraint.

▶ The posterior medial capsule, LCL, and midmedial capsule contributed only modest restraints.

Conclusions

▶ Knee stability and proposed operative procedures should be analyzed in terms of all ligamentous restraints.

▶ Special attention must be given to the primary restraints that cannot be substituted for by the secondary restraints.

▶ Secondary restraints may obscure clinical laxity tests, but these often stretch out and do not provide knee stability under higher activity forces.

▶ The ACL and PCL provide the major resistance to anterior and posterior tibial displacements.

▶ Because of limited secondary restraints, following cruciate injury there is a high risk of altered joint function since functional stability is dependent on muscle restraints and joint geometry.

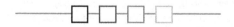

FEATURED ARTICLE

Authors: Hughston JC, Andrews JR, Cross MJ, Mischi A.

Title: Classification of knee ligament instabilities. Part I. The medial compartment and cruciate ligaments.

Journal Information: *J Bone Joint Surg Am.* 1976;58:159–172.

A Top 100 Cited Articles in Clinical Orthopedic Sports Medicine

▸ The authors present a standardized terminology and classification of knee ligament instability based on the clinical and operative findings in 68 knees with acute tears of the medial compartment and cruciate ligaments.

▸ The authors present a detailed description of various knee clinical examination tests:

▷ Abduction stress test

▷ Adduction stress test

▷ Anterior drawer test

▷ Posterior drawer test

▷ "Jerk" test

▷ Recurvatum test

▷ External rotation-recurvatum test

Results

▸ Knee instability is classified into the following categories:

▷ Straight instability (no rotation of the tibia with respect to the femur)

≫ Medial instability

≫ Lateral instability

≫ Posterior instability

≫ Anterior instability

▷ Rotatory instability

≫ Anteromedial rotatory instability

≫ Anterolateral rotatory instability

≫ Posterolateral rotatory instability

≫ Combined rotatory instabilities

⟩ Various combinations of the rotatory instabilities may occur

⟩ Combined anterolateral and posterolateral rotatory instability

⟩ Combined anterolateral and anteromedial rotatory instability

Conclusions

▶ Complete disruption of the medial compartment can occur without subsequent significant pain, effusion, or difficulty walking.

▶ Localized edema and tenderness after injury are good indicators of the site of MCL disruption.

▶ The abduction stress test with the knee at 30 degrees of flexion is completely reliable as an indicator of a complete MCL tear.

▶ A positive abduction stress test at full extension is the most reliable indication of an acute rupture of the PCL in association with medial compartment disruption.

▶ The posterior drawer sign is an unreliable test for an acute PCL rupture, but is always positive in the presence of a chronic PCL rupture.

▶ A strongly positive anterior drawer sign with the tibia in external rotation indicates that the medial capsular, posterior oblique, and ACL are ruptured.

▶ A mildly or moderately positive anterior drawer sign with the tibia in external rotations tells nothing about the ACL, but indicates that the posterior oblique and medial capsular ligaments are torn.

▶ Anteromedial rotatory instability can be recognized by the presence of a positive anterior drawer sign with the tibia externally rotated and a positive abduction stress test with the knee at 30 degrees of flexion.

▶ In the acute stage, increased recurvatum is commonly associated with ACL rupture and not with PCL disruption.

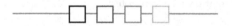

FEATURED ARTICLE

Authors: Hughston JC, Andrews JR, Cross MJ, Mischi A.

Title: Classification of knee ligament instabilities. Part 2. The lateral compartment.

Journal Information: *J Bone Joint Surg Am.* 1976;58:173–179.

▶ The authors classify 6 types of lateral instability of the knee:
▷ Anterolateral rotatory instability
▷ Posterolateral rotatory instability
▷ Combined anterolateral and posterolateral rotatory instability

▷ Combined anterolateral and anteromedial rotatory instability
▷ Combined posterolateral, anterolateral, and anteromedial rotatory instability
▷ Straight lateral instability

Results

▶ Lateral instability of the knee is less frequent but more disabling than medial instability of a comparable amount.

▶ The diagnostic tests for lateral instability are more subtle and more frequently misinterpreted.

▶ Posterolateral rotatory subluxation
▷ This is demonstrated by either an apparently positive posterior drawer test with the tibia in neutral rotation or by the external rotation-recurvatum test with the knee in extension.

▶ Anterolateral rotatory subluxation
▷ The anterior drawer test with the tibia in neutral rotation demonstrates that the lateral tibial condyle appears to become more prominent or that both condyles appear to become equally prominent.
▷ Confirmed by the "jerk" test: a jerk elicited at about 30 degrees of knee flexion as the moderately internally rotated tibia is straightened from 90 degrees of flexion to full extension while a mild abduction stress is applied.

▶ Combined anterolateral and posterolateral rotatory instability.
▷ Characterized by a positive anterior drawer test and apparently positive posterior drawer test.
▷ Adduction stress test that is 1+ or 2+ at 30 degrees of flexion.
▷ Positive external rotation-recurvatum and jerk tests.

▶ Straight lateral instability
▷ Positive adduction stress test at full extension without associated external rotation and recurvatum of the tibia.
▷ Present when the lateral-compartment ligaments are completely torn with an associated PCL tear.

Conclusions

▶ Instabilities due to tears of the lateral-compartment ligaments of the knee are less common but more easily overlooked and are more disabling than the instabilities caused by lesions of the medial-compartment ligaments.

▶ The adduction stress test, usually considered to be pathognomonic of lateral-compartment instabilities, is likely to be only 1+ or 2+ in all types of lateral instability, and is generally not diagnostic.

▶ A negative adduction stress test does not exclude lateral instability.

▶ The "jerk" test is the most specific test for anterolateral rotatory instability.

▶ Posterolateral rotatory instability due to a tear of the arcuate complex is demonstrated most accurately by the external rotation-recurvatum test.

▶ Posterolateral rotatory instability can be missed entirely as the cause of posterolateral joint pain or misdiagnosed as a tear of the lateral meniscus, leading to meniscectomy with resulting increased disability.

▶ It is most important to carefully evaluate knee injuries that may be associated with lateral-compartment ligament tears and to identify the objective signs of lateral instability, which are indications for surgical repair.

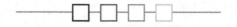

FEATURED ARTICLE

Authors: Gollehon DL, Torzilli PA, Warren RF.

Title: The role of the posterolateral and cruciate ligaments in the stability of the human knee: a biomechanical study.

Journal Information: *J Bone Joint Surg Am*. 1987;69:233–242.

Study Design: Cadaveric Study

▶ Seventeen cadaveric specimens.

▶ Mechanical testing apparatus that allowed 5 degrees of freedom.

▶ Performed selective section of the following:

▷ LCL

▷ Popliteus-arcuate (deep) ligament complex

▷ ACL

▷ PCL

▶ Tested at knee flexion angles ranging from 0 to 90 degrees.

Results

▶ At all flexion angles, the LCL and deep ligament complex functioned together as the principal structures preventing varus rotation and external rotation of the tibia.

▶ At all angles of flexion, the PCL was the principal structure preventing posterior translation.

▶ At flexion angles ≤30 degrees, the amount of posterior translation after sectioning of only the LCL and the deep structures was similar to that seen after isolated PCL sectioning.

▶ Isolated PCL sectioning did not affect varus or external rotation of the tibia at any position of knee flexion.

▶ When the PCL was sectioned after LCL and deep ligament complex sectioning, there was a large increase in posterior translation and varus rotation at all flexion angles.

▶ At flexion angles > 30 degrees, external rotation of the tibia was increased.

▶ Application of internal tibial torque resulted in no increase in tibial rotation after isolated ACL sectioning or combined LCL and deep ligament complex sectioning.

▶ Combined sectioning of all 3 structures increased internal rotation at flexion of 30 and 60 degrees.

▶ The increases in external rotation produced by sectioning the LCL and deep ligament complex were not changed with additional ACL sectioning.

Clinical Relevance

▶ The posterolateral ligaments are important in the prevention of posterior translation, varus rotation, and external tibial rotation.

▶ These findings may also help explain the wide variability of knee function in patients who have injured the ACL or the PCL.

▶ Since the PCL is most functional at greater flexion angles, patients with an isolated injury of that ligament may maintain fairly good knee function in positions closer to extension.

▶ Patients with combined posterolateral and PCL injuries may have knee instability at 0 and 30 degrees with impaired knee function in these positions.

▶ Combined injury of the ACL and posterolateral ligaments may allow enough increased internal and external rotation of the tibia to further impair knee function.

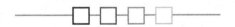

FEATURED ARTICLE

Authors: Noyes FR, Butler DL, Grood ES, Zernicke RF.

Title: Biomechanical analysis of human ligament grafts used in knee-ligament repairs and reconstructions.

Journal Information: *J Bone Joint Surg Am.* 1984;66:344–352.

Study Design: Cadaveric Study

- Tested 90 specimens obtained at autopsy from 18 young people (mean age 26 years, std. dev. 6 years), 14 men, 4 women.
- The purpose of the study was to determine the structural mechanical properties of 9 graft tissues commonly used in ligament reconstructions.
- Different tissue tested:
  - ACL tendon
  - Bone-patellar tendon-bone (central and medial)
  - Semitendinosus
  - Fascia lata
  - Distal iliotibial tract
  - Quadriceps tendon-patellar retinaculum-patellar tendon (medial, central, and lateral)
- Tissues were subjected to high strain-rate failure tests to determine their strength and elongation properties.
- The results were compared with the mechanical properties of ACLs from similar young-adult donors.

Results

Strength

- The bone-patellar tendon bone graft (14 to 15 mm, central or medial portion) was the strongest, with a mean strength of 159% to 168% of the ACL.
- Some graft tissues used in ligament reconstructions are markedly weak and therefore at risk for elongation and failure at low forces.
- Grafts using prepatellar retinacular tissues (14% to 21% strength of ACL) or a narrow width of fascia lata (16% strength of ACL) or distal iliotibial tract (44% strength of ACL) are included in this at-risk group.
- Wider grafts from the iliotibial tract or fascia lata have proportionally increased ultimate strength that can reach that of the ACL.

▶ Semitendinosus tendons have a mean strength of 70% of the ACL.
▶ Gracilis tendons have a mean strength of 49% of the ACL.

Stiffness

▶ Patellar tendon-bone units were 3 to 4 times stiffer than similarly gripped ACLs.
▶ Gracilis and semitendinosus tendon preparations had values that were nearly identical to those of ACLs.
▶ Fascia lata and patellar retinacular graft tissues had much lower stiffnesses than the ACL.

Conclusions and Clinical Relevance

▶ Bone-tendon-bone grafts have a distinct theoretical advantage for earlier graft incorporation at the fixation site and higher initial graft strength, thereby allowing earlier knee motion and a shorter period of disuse and immobility.
▶ Weaker grafts that are more apt to fail prematurely than stronger grafts probably require longer post-op protection to allow time for remodeling.
▶ If wider distal iliotibial-tract grafts are used to increase initial strength, iliotibial tract function may be adversely affected.
▶ Tissues of greater width require larger drill holes if bone fixation is used, and therefore may require additional time for bone ingrowth and graft incorporation.

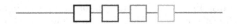

FEATURED ARTICLE

Authors: Warren LF, Marshall JL.

Title: The supporting structures and layers on the medial side of the knee.

Journal Information: *J Bone Joint Surg Am.* 1979;61:56–62.

Study Design: Cadaveric Study

▶ 154 fresh human knee joints were dissected.

- Study goal: To delineate the consistent anatomic structures in the medial side of the knee and to determine their relationship to each other.
- Since definition of the plane of the capsule was fundamental to standardizing the dissections, they first exposed the easily recognizable superficial medial ligament and then the deep medial ligament. The deep ligament was used to define the plane of the capsule, and the limits of the capsule were then determined by blunt dissection.

Results

- A 3-layered pattern was found in which ligaments could be consistently placed.
- Only minor variations in the overall anatomic pattern were found.
- Level I: The "deep fascia" or "crural fascia"
  - ▷ First fascial plane encountered after the skin incision
  - ▷ The sartorius inserts into the network of fascial fibers
- Level II: The "superficial medial ligament"
  - ▷ This plane is clearly defined by the parallel fibers of the superficial medial ligament.
  - ▷ Posteromedial corner
    - » Layer II merges with layer III and with the tendon sheath.
    - » Conjoined structure formed by layers II and III extends posteriorly to form a pouch (posteromedial "capsule") that envelops the medial condyle of the femur.
  - ▷ Semimembranosus tendon
    - » Direct insertion: Most of the tendon inserts in bone through at the posteromedial corner of the tibia just below the joint line.
    - » Anterior insertion: An extension of the direct insertion that lies deep to the superficial medial ligament and layer II, and distal to the tibial margin of the capsule or layer III.
  - ▷ Semimembranosis tendon sheath
    - » Sends fibrous extension upward and downward into layer II, along with a smaller extension that runs distally to insert on the tibia posterior to the inferior oblique portion of the superficial medial ligament.
- Level III: The capsule of the knee joint
  - ▷ Layer III can be separated from all superficial structures except toward the margin of the patella.
  - ▷ Beneath the superficial medial ligament, this layer becomes thicker and forms a vertically oriented band of short fibers known as the deep medial ligament, or medial capsular ligament.
  - ▷ The meniscotibial ligament (coronary ligament) is consistently readily separated from the overlying superficial ligament.

Summary

▸ This paper includes 7 excellent diagrams that illustrate the anatomic structures on the medial side of the knee.

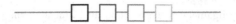

FEATURED ARTICLE

Authors: Seebacher JR, Inglis AE, Marshall JL, Warren RF.

Title: The structure of the posterolateral aspect of the knee.

Journal Information: *J Bone Joint Surg Am.* 1982;64:536–541.

Study Design: Cadaveric Study

▸ 35 cadaveric knees dissected.

Results

▸ The lateral structures of the knee can be divided into 3 distinct layers.
▸ Layer I (most superficial layer)
  ▹ 2 parts.
  ▹ Iliotibial tract and its expansion anteriorly.
  ▹ Superficial portion of the biceps and its expansion posteriorly.
  ▹ Layer is most robust where most of the fibers are vertical.
  ▹ Peroneal nerve lies deep to this layer just posterior to the biceps tendon.
▸ Layer II
  ▹ Formed by the quadriceps retinaculum, most of which descends anterolaterally and adjacent to the patella.
  ▹ Posteriorly, this layer is incomplete and is represented by the two patellofemoral ligaments.
▸ Layer III (deepest layer)
  ▹ Lateral part of the joint capsule, which attaches to the edges of the tibia and femur circumferentially in horizontal planes at the proximal and distal ends of the knee joint.

- ▷ Divides into 2 laminae just posterior to the overlying iliotibial tract.
  - ≫ These laminae encompass 3 ligaments.
    - ⟩ LCL
    - ⟩ Fabellofibular ligament
    - ⟩ Arcuate ligament
- ▷ Coronary ligament is the capsular attachment to the outer edge of the lateral meniscus.
- ▷ Popliteus tendon passes through a hiatus in the coronary ligament to attach to the femur.
- ▶ Layers I and II are adherent to each other in a vertical line at the lateral margin of the patella.
- ▶ Three major anatomic variations of layer III:
  - ▷ Reinforcement of the capsule by the arcuate ligament alone (13%).
  - ▷ Reinforcement of the capsule by the fabellofibular ligament alone (20%).
  - ▷ Reinforcement of the capsule by both ligaments (67%).
  - ▷ The variation pattern can be predicted based on x-ray and physical exam.
    - ≫ When the fabella is seen on x-ray, the fabellofibular ligament will be found deep between the biceps tendon and gastrocnemius lateral head.
    - ≫ Absence of the ossicle indicates that the arcuate ligament will be robust.
    - ≫ When the fabella is invisible on x-ray but can be palpated (cartilaginous fabella), both the fabellofibular and the arcuate ligaments will be present, but they will be smaller than when only one of the two is present.

Summary

- ▶ This paper includes 4 excellent diagrams that illustrate the anatomic structures of the posterolateral aspect of the knee.

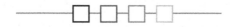

FEATURED ARTICLE

Authors: Arnoczky SP, Warren RF.

Title: Microvasculature of the human meniscus.

Journal Information: *Am J Sports Med*. 1982;10:90–95.

Study Design: Cadaveric Study

▶ 20 cadaveric specimens.

▶ Popliteal artery cannulated and 200 mm of India ink injected.

▶ 10 specimens were frozen and 5 cut into 5-mm-thick sagittal sections and 5 cut into 5-mm-thick coronal sections and then decalcified and cleared using a modified Spalteholz technique.

▶ The menisci of 10 specimens were dissected out en bloc, taking care to preserve the perimeniscal tissues. The menisci were serially sectioned in the transverse plane and alternate sections were processed for either histologic evaluation or tissue clearing.

Results

▶ Vascular supply to the meniscus originates predominantly from the lateral genicular arteries (both inferior and superior).

▶ Branches of these vessels give rise to a perimeniscal capillary plexus within the synovium and capsule that supplies the peripheral 10% to 25% of the meniscus.

▶ The perimeniscal vessels are predominantly oriented in a circumferential pattern with radial branches directed toward the joint center.

▶ The middle genicular artery, along with a few terminal branches of the medial and lateral genicular arteries, supplies vessels to the menisci through the vascular synovium that covers the anterior and posterior horns.

▶ This synovial covering appears continuous with the vascular synovial sheath surrounding the cruciate ligaments.

▶ A peripheral, vascular, synovial fringe extends a short distance over both the femoral and tibial surfaces of the menisci but does not contribute any vessels to the meniscus.

▶ The posterolateral aspect of the lateral meniscus adjacent to the popliteal tendon is lacking any penetrating peripheral vessels or synovial fringe.

Conclusion

▶ Isolated lesions in the inner three-fourths of the meniscus lack the blood supply necessary for an inflammatory and reparative response.

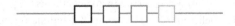

FEATURED ARTICLE

Authors: Ferretti M, Ekdahl M, Shen W, Fu FH.

Title: Osseous landmarks of the femoral attachment of the anterior cruciate ligament: an anatomic study.

Journal Information: *Arthroscopy.* 2007;23:1218–1225.

Study Design: Cadaveric Study

▶ The femoral attachment of the ACL was studied to determine its osseous landmarks with reference to its 2 bundles: the anteromedial and posterolateral bundle.
▶ Studied in 3 settings:
  ▷ Histologic examination in 7 human fetuses.
  ▷ Arthroscopic examination in 60 patients undergoing ACL surgery.
  ▷ Gross examination in 16 cadaveric knees.
    ≫ 3-D laser digitizer pictures of the cadaveric specimens were taken to quantify length, area, and angulations of the femoral attachment of the ACL.

Results

▶ Two different osseous landmarks were detected.
  ▷ An osseous ridge (named the *lateral intercondylar ridge*) that runs from the proximal to distal ends.
    ≫ It was present in all the arthroscopic patients and cadaveric knees.
  ▷ An osseous landmark (named the *lateral bifurcate ridge*) that runs between the femoral attachment of the anteromedial and posterolateral bundles running from anterior to posterior.
    ≫ It was present in 6/7 fetuses, 49/60 arthroscopic patients, and 13/16 cadaveric knees.
▶ A change of slope between the femoral attachment of the anteromedial and posterolateral bundles was observed in all specimens.
▶ The femoral attachment of the anteromedial bundle formed an angle with the posterolateral bundle of 27.6 degrees ± 8.8 degrees and a radius of curvature of 25.7 ± 12 mm.
▶ The area of the entire ACL footprint was 196.8 ± 23.1 mm^2.
▶ The area of the anteromedial bundle was 120 ± 19 mm^2.
▶ The area of the posterolateral bundle was 76.8 ± 15 mm^2.

Conclusions

▶ The ACL femoral attachment has a unique topography.

  ▷ There is a constant presence of the lateral intercondylar ridge.

  ▷ There is often an osseous ridge, the lateral bifurcate ridge, between the anteromedial and postcrolateral bundle femoral attachment.

▶ These landmarks can guide surgeons performing ACL reconstruction in a more anatomic fashion using a double-bundle technique.

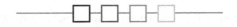

FEATURED ARTICLE
Authors: Tegner Y, Lysholm J.
Title: Rating systems in the evaluation of knee ligament injuries.
Journal Information: *Clin Orthop Relat Res.* 1985;198:43–49.
A Top 100 Cited Articles in Clinical Orthopedic Sports Medicine

Study Design: Cohort Study

▶ This article includes details of the Lysholm knee scoring system and provides a 10-point Tegner and Lysholm activity grading scale.

▶ Studied 76 patients with ACL injury.

▶ The object was to analyze differences between different types of knee rating scores.

  ▷ Lysholm knee scoring scale.

    » A discrete rating scale with 100-point maximum.

  ▷ Marshall scoring system.

    » Includes symptoms, activity grading, results of simple functional tests, and clinical findings with a 50-point maximum.

    » Many items in the Marshall system are graded in a binary fashion (yes/no).

  ▷ Activity score (Tegner and Lysholm).

- Lysholm knee scoring scale
  - ▷ Limp (5 points)
  - ▷ Need for cane/crutch (5 points)
  - ▷ Locking (15 points)
  - ▷ Instability (25 points)
  - ▷ Pain (25 points)
  - ▷ Swelling (10 points)
  - ▷ Stair climbing (10 points)
  - ▷ Squatting (5 points)
- The authors present a new activity grading scale to complement the knee functional score.
  - ▷ Work and sport activities graded numerically from 0 to 10.
  - ▷ 0 = Disability due to knee problem.
  - ▷ 1 to 5 = Work score based on labor demands from sedentary to heavy labor.
  - ▷ 3 to 10 = Increasing sport activity from recreational to competitive sports, based in part on cutting/pivoting involved.
    - » For instance, competitive swimming is scored a 3, while competitive soccer is scored a 10.

Results

- There was significant correlation between scores on the Lysholm knee scoring scale and the Marshall scoring system ($r = 0.78$, $p < 0.001$).
- More patients had excellent/good knee function rating using the Lysholm score.
- Significant differences in Lysholm scores were seen with different activity grading scale scores.
  - ▷ Mean Lysholm of patients with activity level 5 to 10 was 83 ± 10.
  - ▷ Mean Lysholm of patients with activity level 0 was 53 ± 16 ($p < 0.001$).
  - ▷ Only 17% of patients with activity levels 0 to 3 had a Lysholm score > 83.

Conclusions

- Stability testing, functional knee score, performance test, and activity grading are all important in evaluating knee ligament injuries.
- The relative importance of each component varies during the course of treatment and during the follow-up period.

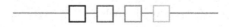

FEATURED ARTICLE

Authors: Lysholm J, Gillquist J.

Title: Evaluation of knee ligament surgery results with special emphasis on use of a scoring scale.

Journal Information: *Am J Sports Med.* 1982;10:150–154.

A Top 100 Cited Articles in Clinical Orthopedic Sports Medicine

Study Design: Cohort Study

▸ The authors developed a scoring scale for knee ligament surgery follow-up.

▸ They added evaluation of instability, which was defined as "giving way" during activity, to the Oretorp modification of the Larson scale.

▸ They compared their scoring scale with the modified Larson scale in 4 groups of patients.

  ▷ Patients with knee ligament injury and anteromedial, anterolateral, or combined anteromedial and anterolateral rotatory instability.

  ▷ Patients with knee ligament injury and posterolateral rotatory or straight posterior instability.

  ▷ Patients with meniscal tears.

  ▷ Patients with chondromalacia patellae.

Results

▸ The 2 scales gave similar results in patients with meniscal tears.

▸ In patients with unstable knees, the new scale gave a significantly lower total score.

▸ The new scale evaluates functional impairment due to clinical instability better than the modified Larson scale.

▸ The new scale total score corresponded to the patients' own opinion of function.

▸ The new scale total score corresponded to the presence or absence of signs of instability.

▸ The reproducibility of their new scoring scale was good.

Lysholm Scoring Scale

- Limp (5 points)
  - ▷ None 5
  - ▷ Slight or periodic 3
  - ▷ Severe and constant 0
- Support (5 points)
  - ▷ Full support 5
  - ▷ Stick or crutch 3
  - ▷ Weight bearing impossible 0
- Stair climbing (10 points)
  - ▷ No problems 10
  - ▷ Slightly impaired 6
  - ▷ 1 step at a time 2
  - ▷ Unable 0
- Squatting (5 points)
  - ▷ No problems 5
  - ▷ Slightly impaired 4
  - ▷ Not past 90 degrees 2
  - ▷ Unable 0
- Walking, running, jumping (70 points)
  - ▷ A: Instability
    - ≫ Never giving way 30
    - ≫ Rarely during athletic or other severe exertion ... 25
    - ≫ Frequently during athletic or other severe exertion (or unable to participate) ... 20
    - ≫ Occasionally in daily activities 10
    - ≫ Often in daily activities 5
    - ≫ Every step 0
  - ▷ B: Pain
    - ≫ None 30
    - ≫ Inconstant and slight during severe exertion ... 25
    - ≫ Marked on giving way 20
    - ≫ Marked during severe exertion 15
    - ≫ Marked on or after walking > 2 km 10
    - ≫ Marked on or after walking < 2 km 5
    - ≫ Constant and severe 0

- Atrophy of thigh (5 points)
  - ▷ None 5
  - ▷ 1 to 2 cm 3
  - ▷ >2 cm 0

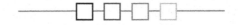

FEATURED ARTICLE

Authors: Engelhart L, Nelson L, Lewis S, Mordin M, Demuro-Mercon C, Uddin S, McLeod L, Cole B, Farr J.

Title: Validation of the Knee Injury and Osteoarthritis Outcome Score subscales for patients with articular cartilage lesions of the knee.

Journal Information: *Am J Sports Med*. 2012;40:2264–2272.

Study Design: Cohort Study

- The Knee Injury and Osteoarthritis Outcome Score (KOOS) was designed to assess acute and chronic knee injuries or early-onset osteoarthritis in young, active patients.
- The KOOS consists of 42 items that cover 5 patient-relevant dimensions (subscales).
  - ▷ Symptoms (7 items)
  - ▷ Pain (9 items)
  - ▷ Activities of daily living (17 items)
  - ▷ Sports/recreation (5 items)
  - ▷ Knee-related quality of life (4 items)
  - ▷ Each subscale is scored from 0 to 100 on a worst-to-best scale.
- This study used both qualitative and quantitative research to evaluate the validity of KOOS subscales among patients with articular cartilage lesions.
- Qualitative analysis
  - ▷ Cognitive interviews, including concept elicitation and cognitive debriefing with the KOOS items, were conducted in 15 patients who were either candidates for cartilage repair or had undergone cartilage repair ≥6 months prior to the study.

- ▶ Quantitative analysis
  - ▷ Psychometric evaluation was conducted with clinical trial data from 54 patients evaluating the Cartilage Autograft Implantation System.
  - ▷ Data collected before surgery and at 7 postsurgical visits up to 12 months.
  - ▷ Assessed internal consistency, test-retest reliability (assessed using data from months 2 and 3), construct validity, responsiveness, and estimates of minimal detectable change.

Results

- ▶ Qualitative research confirmed that the concepts measured on the KOOS are important to patients with articular cartilage lesions, with most participants finding it comprehensive and appropriate.
- ▶ The KOOS subscales had excellent internal consistency reliability (0.74 to 0.97 at baseline).
- ▶ The KOOS subscales had excellent test-retest reliability (0.78 to 0.82).
- ▶ Construct validity findings supported the hypothesized relationships with significant correlations ($r \geq 0.50$) in the expected directions.
- ▶ Responsiveness analyses demonstrated excellent sensitivity to change.
- ▶ Standardized response means ranged from 0.8 to 1.2.
- ▶ Minimal detectable change estimates ranged from 7.4 to 12.1.

Conclusion

- ▶ This study supports the use of the KOOS subscales in patients with articular cartilage lesions.

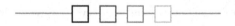

FEATURED ARTICLE
Authors: Irrgang JJ, Anderson AF, Boland AL, Harner CD, Kurosaka M, Neyret P, Richmond JC, Shelborne KD.
Title: Development and validation of the International Knee Documentation Committee Subjective Knee Form.
Journal Information: *Am J Sports Med.* 2001;29:600–613.

Study Design: Cohort Study

▶ The International Knee Documentation Committee (IKDC) Subjective Knee Form was designed to measure improvement or deterioration in symptoms, function, and sports activity in patients with a variety of knee conditions, including ligament injuries, meniscal injuries, articular cartilage lesions, and patellofemoral pain.

▶ The IKDC Subjective Knee Form was designed to represent symptoms and limitations in function and sports activity due to knee impairment and to maximize test-retest reliability, responsiveness, and validity.

▷ 7 questions on knee symptoms

▷ 2 questions on sports activities

▷ 1 question on knee function prior to injury and at present

▶ Study purpose: To evaluate the reliability and validity of the IKDC Subjective Knee Form.

▶ Administered IKDC Subjective Knee Form and SF-36 to 533 patients with a variety of knee problems.

▶ Analyses performed to determine reliability, validity, and differential item function related to age, sex, and diagnosis.

Results

▶ Factor analysis revealed a single dominant component, making it reasonable to combine all questions into a single score.

▶ Internal consistency was 0.92.

▶ Test-retest reliability was 0.95.

▶ Based on test-retest reliability, the value for a true change in the score was 9 points.

▶ The IKDC Subjective Knee Form score was related to concurrent measures of physical function ($r = 0.47$ to 0.66), but not to emotional function ($r = 0.16$ to 0.26).

▶ Analysis of differential item function indicated that the questions functioned similarly for men vs women, young vs old, and for those with different diagnoses.

Conclusions

▶ The IKDC Subjective Knee Form is a reliable and valid knee-specific measure of symptoms, function, and sports activity.

▶ The IKDC Subjective Knee Form is appropriate for patients with a wide variety of knee problems.

▸ Using the same form for all patients can simplify data collection and permit comparisons of outcomes across groups with different knee problems.

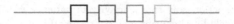

CLASSIC ARTICLE

Authors: Fukubayashi T, Kurosawa H.

Title: The contact area and pressure distribution pattern of the knee. A study of normal and osteoarthritic knee joints.

Journal Information: *Acta Orthop Scand.* 1980;51:871–879.

Study Design: Cadaveric Study

▸ 7 fresh frozen knees studied.
▸ Contact area and pressure distribution measured.
▸ Contact areas measured before and after meniscectomy under loads of 200 N, 500 N, and 1000 N.
▸ Fiji film used to directly measure pressure distribution.

Results

▸ Contact area increased as the load increased.
▸ Contact area before meniscus removal was more than twice as large as after meniscus removal.
▸ Medial compartment contact area was always larger than the lateral compartment, but as the load increased, this difference gradually decreased.
▸ At a load of 1000 N, the knee contact area was 1150 mm^2 with menisci and 520 mm^2 without menisci, and the menisci occupied 70% of the total contact area.
▸ Peak pressure at 1000 N was 3 MPa with the menisci and 6 MPa without them.
▸ High-pressure areas were located on the lateral meniscus and on the uncovered part of the articular cartilage of the lateral compartment and on the uncovered cartilage in the medial compartment.
▸ After removal of the menisci, the contact area decreased to below one half that of the intact knee and the contact pressure considerably increased.

▸ Contact areas measured in two osteoarthritic knees were significantly larger than those in normal knees.

Conclusions

▸ These facts imply that the menisci have load-bearing and load-spreading functions.

▸ In arthritic knees, the menisci seemed to play a less significant role in the transmission of weight than in normal knees.

Meniscal Tear Debridement and Repair

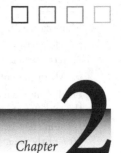

Chapter 2

FEATURED ARTICLE

Authors: Cannon WD, Vittori JM.

Title: The incidence of healing in arthroscopic meniscal repairs in anterior-cruciate ligament reconstructed knees versus stable knees.

Journal Information: *Am J Sports Med.* 1992;20:176–181.

Study Design: Retrospective Review

- Compared the incidence of meniscal repair healing in knees undergoing anterior cruciate ligament (ACL) reconstruction to that in stable knees without ACL injury.
- Reviewed 117 meniscal repairs in 105 patients.
  - 30 (29%) women, 75 (71%) men.
  - 10 bilateral meniscal repairs.
  - 2 patients had a meniscus repaired a second time after failure of the initial repair.
- Follow-up data were obtained in 90 of 117 meniscal repairs.
  - 32 (36%) acute (less than 8 weeks from injury) tears.
  - 58 (64%) chronic meniscal tears.
  - Group I: 68 meniscal repairs in conjunction with ACL reconstruction.
  - Group II: 22 isolated meniscal repairs in ACL stable knees.

Miller MD, Mauffrey C, Hak DJ.
Rapid Reference Review in Sports Medicine:
Pivotal Papers Revealed (pp 27-39).
© 2016 Taylor & Francis Group.

▸ Meniscal healing was assessed by either arthroscopy or arthrography.

▷ Mean time of assessment 10 months for repairs done with ACL reconstruction.

▷ Mean time of assessment 7 months for isolated repairs.

▸ Healed meniscus = healed over the length of the tear with a residual cleft at the tear site of less than 10% of the meniscal thickness.

▸ Incompletely healed menisci = a residual cleft at the tear site of less than 50% of the meniscal thickness.

▸ Failed healing = residual cleft > 50% of the meniscal thickness at any location along the tear site.

Results

▸ 82% overall rate of successful healing

▷ 93% rate of successful healing in group I (with ACL reconstruction).

▷ 50% rate of successful healing in group II (stable knees) ($P < 0.00005$).

▸ Tear length and healing rate

▷ 94% successful healing (complete or incomplete) in tear lengths < 2 cm.

▷ 86% successful healed (complete or incomplete) in tear lengths of 2 to 4 cm.

▷ 50% successful healing (complete or incomplete) in tear lengths > 4 cm.

▸ Lateral vs medial meniscus

▷ Lateral meniscus repairs

≫ 93% overall successful healing rate (complete or incomplete).

≫ 100% successful healing rate (complete or incomplete) in repairs associated with ACL reconstruction.

≫ 70% successful healing rate (complete or incomplete) in isolated repairs.

▷ Medial meniscus repairs

≫ 73% overall successful healing rate (complete or incomplete).

≫ 86% successful healing rate (complete or incomplete) in repairs associated with ACL reconstruction.

≫ Only 34% successful healing rate (complete or incomplete) in isolated repairs.

▸ Healing rate by age group

▷ 54% successful healing (complete or incomplete) in patients ≥ 18 years.

▷ 85% successful healing (complete or incomplete) in patients 19 to 22 years.

▷ 86% successful healing (complete or incomplete) in patients 23 to 30 years.

▷ 89% successful healing (complete or incomplete) in patients 31 to 35 years.

▷ 90% successful healing (complete or incomplete) in patients > 35 years (range 35 to 57 years).

- Acute vs chronic tears.
  - ▷ 88% successful healing (complete or incomplete) in acute tears (within 8 weeks of injury).
  - ▷ 79% successful healing (complete or incomplete) in chronic tears ($P < 0.25$).

Conclusions

- Patients with ACL reconstruction did better than those with isolated meniscal repair, regardless of tear length.
  - ▷ Reasons postulated why these repairs have better healing rates include:
    - » ACL reconstruction protects the meniscal repair from the biomechanical forces during anterior tibial subluxation that originally caused the tear.
    - » ACL surgery causes more intra-articular trauma, producing more bleeding and fibrin clot formation, which provides an important adjunct to the healing process.
    - » Some knees with isolated meniscal tears may have biomechanical abnormalities or an unidentified impairment in joint configuration that predisposes the meniscus to tear initially and predisposes the repaired meniscus to retear.
- Lateral meniscal repairs fared better than medial repairs in both groups.
- Older patients had better healing than younger ones.
- Overall, acute repairs were more successful than repairs of chronic tears.
- However, group 1 (ACL reconstruction) patients with chronic tears still had a 91% successful healing rate.

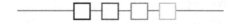

FEATURED ARTICLE

Authors: Hanks GA, Gause TM, Handal JA, Kalenak A.

Title: Meniscus repair in the anterior cruciate deficient knee

Journal Information: *Am J Sports Med.* 1990;18:606–613.

Study Design: Retrospective Review

- Purpose: To evaluate the meniscal repair success rate in an ACL-deficient knee.
- Isolated peripheral vascular zone meniscal tear repairs in 22 patients (23 menisci) with ACL insufficiency who for various reasons did not have an ACL reconstruction/repair.
- Meniscus repair performed by:
  - ▷ Open arthrotomy in 12 cases.
  - ▷ Arthroscopically in 11 cases.
- Average age 25 years (range 15 to 48 years), 4 women, 18 men.
- Average follow-up 56 months.
- 16 patients (with 17 meniscal repairs) returned for an interview and physical examination.
- 6 patients were contacted by telephone, but each of these had been examined at least 2 years post-op.
- Follow-up focused on:
  - ▷ Presence, character, and location of pain.
  - ▷ Presence of swelling.
  - ▷ Whether symptoms of catching, snapping, or locking were present.
  - ▷ Activity level and limitations as measured by Tegner and Lysholm activity scores.
  - ▷ Physical examination.
- Given the length of follow-up, the investigators assumed that the meniscus had healed if there was an absence of any clinical symptoms or physical findings.

Results

- Pain
  - ▷ 6 patients (26%) had mild occasional pain not requiring medication.
  - ▷ 1 patient had moderate pain requiring nonnarcotic pain medication.

- Instability
  - ▷ 8 patients (26%) had occasional giving-way episodes, and one underwent ACL reconstruction 5 years later because of frequent giving way.
- Activity level
  - ▷ 9 patients lost one or more grades of the Tegner activity score since their injury.
    - » 4 of these were due to graduation from college or high school, after which they participated only in recreational rather than competitive sports.
    - » 1 patient attempted to return to college football, but even though he was not having significant knee symptoms, he was unable to perform at his previous level.
    - » 4 patients had lost at least one grade in the Tegner activity score because of knee symptoms of pain, instability, or both.
- 7 patients underwent repeat arthroscopic examinations.
  - ▷ 4 were found to have healed meniscal lesions.
  - ▷ 3 had meniscal tears at either the previous repair site or more central on the same meniscus.
  - ▷ All new tears, even if they occurred at another site of the same meniscus, were rated as failures.
- Meniscus repair was successful (in terms of preservation of the meniscus) in 87% of ACL-deficient knees.
- 3 patients (13%) had failed repairs or a retear and required subsequent partial meniscectomy.
- No significant differences between the results of open or arthroscopic repair.

Conclusion

- Meniscus repair is not contraindicated in an ACL-deficient knee even though the failure rate of meniscus repair may be greater in an unstable knee.

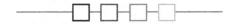

FEATURED ARTICLE

Authors: Johnson RJ, Kettelkamp DB, Clark W, Leaverton P.

Title: Factors affecting late results after meniscectomy.

Journal Information: *J Bone Joint Surg Am.* 1974;56:719–729.

Study Design: Retrospective Review

▶ Review of patients who underwent meniscectomy at University of Iowa between 1927 and 1964.

▶ Exclusion criteria: Rheumatoid arthritis, osteochondritis dissecans, knees with greater than "very slight laxity," patients who underwent bilateral meniscectomies.

▶ 99 patients who had one or both menisci removed from a single knee returned for examination.

  ▷ 74 medial meniscectomies.

  ▷ 19 lateral meniscectomies.

  ▷ 6 both medial and lateral meniscectomies.

  ▷ Only 7 patients had minor x-ray changes at the time of their meniscectomy.

▶ Mean age at time of surgery 27.1 years, 76 men, 23 women.

▶ Average follow-up 17.5 years (5 to 37 years).

▶ Clinical rating system

  ▷ Activity level (ranging from walking only with support to unrestricted running and jumping).

  ▷ Pain with activity (ranging from pain with any weight bearing to no pain with the most vigorous activities).

  ▷ Pain with reinjury

  ▷ Effusion

  ▷ Giving way

  ▷ Catching

  ▷ Ability to climb stairs

  ▷ Ability to walk on rough ground

  ▷ Ability to squat

  ▷ Ability to return to sports activities.

  ▷ Each item was designated as excellent, good, fair, or poor.

  ▷ Final knee rating was the lowest rating assigned to any of the 10 criteria.

▶ X-rays were made of both knees at the time of follow-up.

  ▷ Evaluated without knowledge of which meniscus had been removed.

▷ Measured cartilage spaces in all 3 compartments.
  » Normal
  » Narrowed less than half the normal thickness
  » Narrowed more than half the normal thickness
  » Obliterated
▷ Osteophytes were recorded according to location and size on a scale of 1 to 5.

Results

▸ 42.5% Satisfactory outcome (excellent or good rating).
▸ 57.5% Unsatisfactory outcome (fair or poor rating).
  ▷ 27 knees rated excellent
  ▷ 15 knees rated good
  ▷ 36 knees rated fair
  ▷ 21 knees rated poor
▸ The longer the duration of symptoms and the greater the frequency of reinjuries (effusion, giving way, and locking) before meniscectomy, the worse the final result (P=0.001).
  ▷ Mean duration of symptoms preoperatively
    » 22.3 months in the group with excellent results.
    » 24.1 months in the group with good results.
    » 39.1 months in the group with fair results.
    » 39.6 months in the group with poor results.
▸ Results were better after medial than after lateral meniscectomy, and worst after removal of both menisci.
▸ Ligamentous laxity, including anteromedial rotational instability, was associated with a poor recovery rating.
▸ Women tended to have a poorer recovery rating than men ($P = 0.04$).
▸ X-rays showed an increase in the frequency of cartilage-space narrowing in the compartment where the meniscectomy had been performed, compared to other compartments in the same knee and in the contralateral knee ($P = 0.001$).
▸ 74% of knees following meniscectomy showed at least one of Fairbank's changes, whereas only 6% of the contralateral knees had such changes.
▸ The frequency of unsatisfactory results increased as the number of Fairbank's changes found in the knees increased ($P = 0.001$).

Conclusions

▸ The authors concluded that the high incidence of abnormal physical and x-ray findings after meniscectomy suggests that the meniscus has important physiological and biomechanical functions.

▶ They cautioned that meniscectomy is not a procedure that can be considered lightly, since the loss of the meniscus is followed by significant morbidity.

▶ They indicated the need to define more precisely the physiological and bio-mechanical functions of the meniscus.

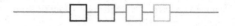

FEATURED ARTICLE

Authors: Sihvonen R, Paavola M, Malmivaara A, Itälä A, Joukainen A, Nurmi H, Kalske J, Järvinen TL, Finnish Degenerative Meniscal Lesion Study (FIDELITY) Group.

Title: Arthroscopic partial meniscectomy versus sham surgery for a degenerative meniscal tear.

Journal Information: *N Engl J Med.* 2013;369(26):2515–2524.

Study Design: Prospective Randomized Study

▶ Multicenter, randomized, double-blind, sham-controlled study.

▶ 146 patients ages 35 to 65 years who had knee symptoms consistent with a degenerative medial meniscus tear and no knee osteoarthritis.

▶ Preop magnetic resonance imaging (MRI) was performed to confirm the medial meniscus tear, but the eligibility of the patients was ultimately determined by arthroscopic examination.

▶ Treatment randomized to arthroscopic partial meniscectomy or sham surgery.

▶ A standard arthroscopic partial meniscectomy was simulated for the sham surgery. After undergoing a standard diagnostic arthroscopy, a standard procedure was followed to mimic the sensations and sounds of a partial meniscectomy. The surgeon asked for all instruments and manipulated the knee as if an arthroscopic partial meniscectomy was being performed. The patient was kept in the operating room for the amount of time required to perform an actual arthroscopic partial meniscectomy.

▶ Outcome measurements at 12 months

▷ Changes in Lysholm score

▷ Changes in Western Ontario Meniscal Evaluation Tool (WOMET) scores

» Each score ranges from 0 to 100, with lower scores indicating more severe symptoms.

▷ Knee pain after exercise (rated from 0 to 10, with 0 indicating no pain).

Results

▶ No significant differences between the 2 treatment groups in the change from baseline to 12 months in any primary outcome in the intention-to-treat analysis.

▶ Mean changes (improvements) in the primary outcome measures:

  ▷ Lysholm score

    » 21.7 points in the partial meniscectomy group

    » 23.3 points in the sham surgery group

    » Between-group difference, −1.6 points; 95% confidence interval [CI], 7.2 to 4.0)

  ▷ WOMET score

    » 24.6 points in the partial meniscectomy group

    » 27.1 points in the sham surgery group

    » Between-group difference, −2.5 points; 95% CI, −9.2 to 4.1

  ▷ Score for knee pain after exercise

    » 3.1 points in the partial meniscectomy group

    » 3.3 points in the sham surgery group

    » Between-group difference, −0.1; 95% CI, −0.9 to 0.7

▶ No significant differences between groups in the number of patients who required subsequent knee surgery.

  ▷ 2 in the partial meniscectomy group

  ▷ 5 in the sham surgery group

▶ No significant differences between groups in serious adverse events.

  ▷ 1 in the partial meniscectomy group

  ▷ None in the sham surgery group

Conclusion

▶ The outcomes after arthroscopic partial meniscectomy were no better than those after a sham surgical procedure in this group of patients ages 35 to 65 with symptoms of a degenerative medial meniscus tear but without knee osteoarthritis.

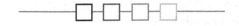

FEATURED ARTICLE

Authors: Miller MD, Ritchie JR, Gomez BA, Royster RM, DeLee JC.

Title: Meniscal repair: an experimental study in the goat.

Journal Information: *Am J Sports Med.* 1995;23:124–128.

Study Design: Animal Study

- Study performed in 24 adult goats
- Longitudinal medial meniscus tear produced in both knees
  - Meniscus repairs in one knee
    - Meniscus repaired with two 2-0 polydioxane (PDS) horizontal mattress sutures using a modified inside-out technique
  - Meniscus left unrepaired in the other knee
- 3 groups of 8 animals each
  - Tear created in peripheral 20% to 25% of meniscus and ACL left intact
  - Tear created in peripheral 40% to 50% of meniscus (in avascular region) and ACL left intact
  - Tear created in peripheral 20% to 15% of meniscus and ACL sectioned
- Animals sacrificed at 6 months post-op
  - Evaluated with arthrogram by blinded observer
  - Meniscus harvested and evaluated by blinded observer
  - Healed menisci evaluated histologically

Results

- Peripheral 20% to 25% tear location with ACL intact (one animal lost prior to 6-month time point)
  - 6/7 repaired menisci healed
  - 1/7 unrepaired menisci healed
- Peripheral 40% to 50% tear location with ACL intact
  - 1/8 repaired menisci healed
  - 0/8 unrepaired menisci healed
- Peripheral 20% to 25% tear location and ACL sections
  - 1/8 repaired menisci healed
  - 0/8 unrepaired menisci healed

▸ Arthrography was 92% accurate in predicting the status of the meniscus repair.

Conclusion

▸ Study supports current clinical practices in meniscal repair and emphasizes the importance of tear location and knee stability in successful meniscal repair.

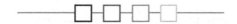

FEATURED ARTICLE
Authors: Cabaud HE, Rodkey WG, Fitzwater JE.
Title: Medial meniscus repairs: an experimental and morphologic study.
Journal Information: *Am J Sports Med.* 1981;9:129–134.

Study Design: Animal Study

▸ Study performed in 20 skeletally mature canines and 12 rhesus monkeys
▸ Anterior horn of the medial meniscus was incised transversely to simulate a deep parrot beak–type laceration
▸ Meniscal tear repaired with a single 3-0 Dexon mattress suture
▸ Limbs immobilized in a cast in 60 degrees flexion for 6 weeks
▸ Animals sacrificed 4 months post-op and menisci examined grossly and excised for histologic examination
▸ Grading of meniscal healing
  ▷ Good = inner meniscal rim was restored without distortion of the remaining meniscus and no degenerative changes.
  ▷ Fair = meniscus had incomplete healing with a defect in the inner rim and some buckling but no degenerative changes.
  ▷ Poor = meniscus had failed to heal and showed a persistent inner rim defect with distortion of the medial meniscus; degenerative changes or articular erosions were associated with the meniscal lesion.

Results

▸ 12/32 (38%) healed completely with restoration of the inner meniscal rim.

▶ 18/32 (56%) showed partial healing sufficient to protect the underlying articular cartilage.

▶ 2/32 (6%) of the menisci failed to heal.

▶ Histology showed that the scar tissue in the meniscal repair was composed of unorganized collagen that lacked normal ground substance.

▶ 10 separate histologic sections were examined for each meniscus, and there was no difference between the scars in the repairs graded as good and fair.

Conclusions

▶ The menisci healed by means of a fibrovascular scar that lacked normal ground substance or organized collagen.

▶ The healed menisci protected the underlying articular surface for the duration of this study.

▶ This study showed that meniscal tears involving the vascular periphery can heal.

▶ The authors concluded that peripheral meniscal tears should be repaired rather than treated by meniscectomy to preserve the integrity, function, and bulk of the medial meniscus to prevent the long-term effects following meniscectomy.

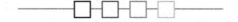

CLASSIC ARTICLE

Author: Fairbank TJ.

Title: Knee joint changes after meniscectomy.

Journal Information: *J Bone Joint Surg Br.* 1948;30:664–670.

A Top 100 Cited Articles in Clinical Orthopedic Sports Medicine

Study Design: Retrospective Review

▶ Reviewed radiographic findings of 107 patients following meniscectomy
  ▷ 80 medial meniscectomies
  ▷ 27 lateral meniscectomies
  ▷ Interval from meniscectomy ranged from 3 months to 14 years

Results

- ▶ Medial meniscectomy patient radiographic findings
  - ▷ 33% no change
  - ▷ 43% ridge formation
  - ▷ 32% joint space narrowing
  - ▷ 18% flattening of the femoral condyle
- ▶ Lateral meniscectomy patient radiographic findings
  - ▷ 50% no change
  - ▷ 7% ridge formation
  - ▷ 40% joint space narrowing
  - ▷ 17% flattening of the femoral condyle
- ▶ They also examined the effect of weight bearing by obtaining non-weight-bearing x-rays in the morning, then obtaining full weight-bearing x-rays, and then obtaining weight-bearing x-rays at the end of the day.
  - ▷ Only a small number of views were identical to allow comparison, but they indicated that the joint space narrowed by 1 mm with weight bearing and by another 1 mm by the end of the day of weight bearing.

Conclusions

- ▶ Identified hallmark changes of early osteoarthritis following meniscectomy
  - ▷ Ridge formation (osteophytes)
  - ▷ Joint-space narrowing
  - ▷ Flattening of the femoral condyle
- ▶ Concluded that these changes were due to the loss of the weight-bearing function of the meniscus
- ▶ Cautioned that meniscectomy is not innocuous

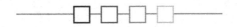

REVIEW ARTICLES

Laible C, Stein DA, Kiridly DN. Meniscal repair. *J Am Acad Orthop Surg.* 2013;21:204–213.

Greis PE, Bardana DD, Holmstrom MC, Burks RT. Meniscus injury: I. Basic science and evaluation. *J Am Acad Orthop Surg.* 2002;10:168–187.

Meniscal Transplantation

Chapter 3

FEATURED ARTICLE

Authors: Noyes FR, Barber-Westin SD, Rankin M.

Title: Meniscal transplantation in symptomatic patients less than fifty years old.

Journal Information: *J Bone Joint Surg Am.* 2004;86:1392–1404.

Study Design: Cohort Study

- 40 meniscal allograft transplants in 38 patients
  - 16 knees also had an osteochondral autograft transfer.
  - 9 knees also had a knee ligament reconstruction.
- Average age at surgery 30 years (14 to 49), 20 men, 18 women
- 37 patients followed for a mean of 40 months (24 to 69 months)
- 1 patient could not return for follow-up, but completed subjective and functional assessment and was interviewed 5 years post-op.
- Outcomes measured:
  - Cincinnati Knee Rating System
  - Symptoms
  - Functional limitations
  - Sports activity level
  - Occupational rating system

Miller MD, Mauffrey C, Hak DJ.
*Rapid Reference Review in Sports Medicine:
Pivotal Papers Revealed (pp 41-48).*
© 2016 Taylor & Francis Group.

▸ Meniscal allograft characteristics were determined with use of a rating system that combined clinical examination (meniscal signs, pain, and clinical symptoms), follow-up arthroscopy (13 patients) and magnetic resonance imaging (MRI) findings (peripheral attachment status, position in joint, signal intensity).

Results

▸ 34 patients (89%) rated their knee as improved.

▸ Mean Cincinnati Knee Rating Scale pain score was 2.5 points (range 0 to 6) preop and improved to a mean of 5.8 points (range 0 to 10) at latest follow-up ($P < 0.0001$).

▸ All patients had knee pain preop, whereas post-op 27 knees (68%) had no pain and 13 (33%) had only mild compartment pain at the latest follow-up.

▸ 30 patients (79%) had pain with daily activities prior to surgery, but only 4 (11%) had such pain at latest follow-up.

▸ Significant improvements were also seen in swelling, walking, stair climbing, squatting, running, jumping, and twisting or turning.

▸ 29 patients (76%) returned to light low-impact sports without problems.

▸ Concomitant osteochondral autograft transfer and knee ligament reconstruction procedures improved knee function and did not increase the rate of complications.

▸ Meniscal allograft characteristics:
  ▷ Normal 17 knees (43%)
  ▷ Altered 12 knees (30%)
  ▷ Failed 11 knees (28%)

Conclusions

▸ Short-term results of meniscal transplantation are promising, as patients show reduced knee pain and increased function.

▸ Long-term outcome of meniscal transplant function and any chondroprotective effect remain unknown and require further investigation.

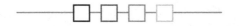

FEATURED ARTICLE

Authors: Cole BJ, Dennis MG, Lee SJ, Nho SJ, Kalsi RS, Hayden JK, Verma NN.

Title: Prospective evaluation of allograft meniscus transplantation: a minimum 2-year follow-up.

Journal Information: *Am J Sports Med.* 2006;34:919–927.

Study Design: Cohort Study

▸ 44 meniscal allograft transplants in 39 patients with a minimum 2-year follow-up.

▸ 4 transplants failed early, leaving 40 transplants in 36 patients for review.

▸ 21 menisci (52.5%) were transplanted in isolation.

▸ 19 menisci (47.5%) transplantations were combined with other procedures for concomitant articular cartilage injury.

▸ Mean age 31 years (16 to 48 years), 22 men, 14 women

▸ Mean follow-up 33.5 months (24 to 57 months)

▸ Outcome measurements:

  ▷ Lysholm score

  ▷ Tegner score

  ▷ International Knee Documentation Committee (IKDC)

  ▷ Knee Injury and Osteoarthritis Outcome Score (KOOS)

  ▷ Noyes symptom rating and sports activity

  ▷ SF-12 score

  ▷ Visual analog pain scales

  ▷ Patient satisfaction

  ▷ Physical examination

Results

▸ Statistically significant improvements from preop scores to final follow-up ($P < 0.05$) in:

  ▷ Lysholm score

  ≫ 52.4 preop

  ≫ 71.6 at the latest follow-up

▷ Tegner score
  ≫ 5 preop
  ≫ 6.5 at the latest follow-up
▷ Noyes sports activity score
  ≫ 58.4 preop
  ≫ 70.9 at the latest follow-up
▷ IKDC score
  ≫ 46.2 preop
  ≫ 64.1 at the latest follow-up
▶ Visual analogue score (VAS) scores also declined significantly from preop to final follow-up for both pain and overall knee condition ($P < 0.05$).
▶ Treatment had failed at final follow-up in 7 patients.
▶ Overall, 77.5% of patients reported they were completely or mostly satisfied with the procedure.
▶ 90% of patients were classified as normal or nearly normal using the IKDC knee examination score at final follow-up.
▶ No significant differences in outcomes of medial menisci transplant vs lateral meniscus transplant, although the lateral transplant group did demonstrate a trend toward greater improvement.
▶ No significant difference between the isolated transplants vs those combined with other procedures.

Conclusions

▶ Meniscus transplantation alone or in combination with other reconstructive procedures results in reliable improvements in knee pain and function at minimum 2-year follow-up.
▶ Although the early clinical results are encouraging, the authors noted that longer-term studies are needed to determine if transplantation can prevent the articular degeneration associated with meniscectomy.

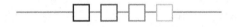

FEATURED ARTICLE

Authors: Verdonk PC, Verstraete KL, Almqvist KF, De Cuyper K, Veys EM, Verbruggen G, Verdonk R.

Title: Meniscal allograft transplantation: long-term clinical results with radiological and magnetic resonance imaging correlations.

Journal Information: *Knee Surg Sports Traumatol Arthrosc.* 2006;14:694–706.

Study Design: Cohort Study

- Long-term review of prospectively collected data
- 42 meniscal allograft transplants in 41 patients with a minimum 10-year follow-up
- 27 medial meniscus transplants
    - 11/27 also had a high tibial osteotomy.
- 15 lateral meniscus transplants
- Outcome measurements:
    - Modified hospital for special surgery (HSS) score
    - KOOS
- Radiographic evaluation in 32 patients
- Magnetic resonance imaging evaluation in 17 patients at about 1 year post-op and at final follow-up
- Patients divided into 3 groups for statistical analysis:
    - Lateral meniscus transplantation
    - Medial meniscus transplantation alone
    - Medial meniscus transplantation with high tibial osteotomy

Results

- 18% overall failure rate
- 7 cases were converted to a total knee arthroplasty during the follow-up period.
- Modified HSS score:
    - Significant improvement in pain and function scores at the final follow-up for all groups
- Medial meniscus transplantation associated with high tibial osteotomy resulted in a greater improvement at the final follow-up compared to medial meniscus transplantation alone.

- The KOOS scores at final follow-up showed the presence of substantial disability, substantial symptoms, and a reduced quality of life.
- Radiographic analysis (available for 32 cases)
  - ▷ 13/32 (40%) knees had no further joint-space narrowing.
  - ▷ 9/32 (28%) knees had no deterioration in Fairbank's changes.
- Magnetic resonance imaging analysis (available in 17 knees):
  - ▷ 6/17 (35%) knees had no progression of cartilage degeneration.
  - ▷ Increased allograft signal intensity and partial graft extrusion were seen in the majority of patients at final follow-up.

Conclusions

- Long-term results after meniscus allograft transplantation are encouraging in terms of pain relief and improvement of function.
- However, substantial disability and symptoms were present in all investigated subgroups.
- Progression of further cartilage degeneration or joint-space narrowing was absent in a considerable number of cases, indicating a potential chondroprotective effect of meniscal transplantation.

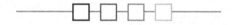

FEATURED ARTICLE
Authors: Wirth CJ, Peters G, Milachowski KA, Weismeier KG, Kohn D.
Title: Long-term results of meniscal allograft transplantation.
Journal Information: *Am J Sports Med*. 2002;30:174–181.

Study Design: Cohort Study

- Long-term prospective study of patients treated with medial meniscal transplantation combined with anterior cruciate ligament (ACL) reconstruction.
- 23 patients
  - ▷ 17 lyophilized meniscal allograft
  - ▷ 6 deep-frozen meniscal allograft
- Average age 29.6 years (21 to 45 years), 20 men, 3 women

- ▶ Outcome measurements:
  - ▷ Clinical assessment
  - ▷ Lysholm score
  - ▷ Radiographs
  - ▷ Magnetic resonance imaging (9 patients)
  - ▷ Second-look arthroscopy (19 patients)
- ▶ All patients evaluated at 3 and 14 years post-op
- ▶ For analysis of long-term results, the study group was compared with 2 control groups that had also undergone ACL reconstruction, with one group having previously undergone meniscectomy and one with intact menisci.

Results

- ▶ Mean Lysholm score:
  - ▷ 59 ± 11 preop
  - ▷ 84 ± 12 at 3 years
  - ▷ 75 ± 21 at 14 years
  - ▷ Statistically significant difference ($P < 0.05$) between patients treated with lyophilized meniscal allograft transplants or patients who had undergone meniscectomy vs the patients with intact menisci or deep-frozen meniscal transplants.
- ▶ Mean Tegner score
  - ▷ 1.0 preop
  - ▷ 5.1 at 3 years
  - ▷ 4.6 at 14 years
- ▶ Patients treated with deep-frozen meniscal transplants generally had better results than patients with lyophilized meniscal transplants.
- ▶ Magnetic resonance imaging showed good preservation of the deep-frozen meniscal transplants, even after 14 years.
- ▶ Lyophilized meniscal transplants were reduced in size at the second-look arthroscopy and on MRI.
- ▶ Comparison to control groups:
  - ▷ Deep-frozen meniscal allografts were found to be more comparable to the control group with an intact meniscus.
  - ▷ Lyophilized meniscal allografts were more comparable with the control group knees that had undergone prior meniscectomy.

Conclusions

- ▶ With both deep-frozen and lyophilized meniscal transplants, there was a deterioration of clinical results during the 14-year follow-up period.
- ▶ Patients with deep-frozen meniscal transplants generally had better results than those treated with lyophilized meniscal transplants.

- Lyophilized meniscal transplants were found to be reduced in size early on, even at the time of second-look arthroscopy (3.8 years) and therefore cannot restore normal meniscus function.
- Cartilage protection is only possible with the deep-frozen meniscal transplants.
- Long-term follow-up results are affected by the initial cartilage condition.
- Graft versus host reaction or disease transmission has not been a problem in any patient.

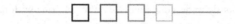

REVIEW ARTICLES

Brophy RH, Matava MJ. Surgical options for meniscal replacement. *J Am Acad Orthop Surg.* 2012;20:265–272.

Packer JD, Rodeo SA. Meniscal allograft transplantation. *Clin Sports Med.* 2009;28:259–283.

□ □ ▢ ▢

Osteochondral Lesions

Chapter **4**

Study Design: Animal Study

▶ Investigated the biologic effect of continuous passive motion on healing of a full-thickness articular cartilage defect in rabbits

  ▷ 3 treatment groups

   » Continuous passive motion (CPM)

   » Intermittent motion (normal cage activity)

   » Immobilization

▶ A full-thickness defect was made in 4 standard sites:

  ▷ Patellar groove

  ▷ Anterior aspect of medial femoral condyle

  ▷ Middle aspect of medial femoral condyle

  ▷ Middle aspect of lateral femoral condyle

▶ 480 defects in the knees of 120 adolescent rabbits

Miller MD, Mauffrey C, Hak DJ.
Rapid Reference Review in Sports Medicine:
Pivotal Papers Revealed (pp 49-66).
© 2016 Taylor & Francis Group.

- 108 defects in the knees of 27 adult rabbits
- Healing of defects assessed weekly:
  - ▷ Gross examination
  - ▷ Light microscopy
    - » Nature of reparative tissue
    - » Degree of metachromasia of the matrix as demonstrated by toluidine-blue staining

Results

- Metaplasia of the healing tissue within the defects from undifferentiated mesenchymal tissue to hyaline articular cartilage was both much more rapid and more complete in animals treated with CPM.
- Rate of healing with hyaline cartilage in adolescent rabbits at 3 weeks:
  - ▷ 8% in immobilized group
  - ▷ 9% in intermittent motion group
  - ▷ 52% in CPM group
- Rate of healing with hyaline cartilage in adult rabbits at 3 weeks:
  - ▷ 3% in immobilized group
  - ▷ 5% in intermittent motion group
  - ▷ 44% in CPM group

Paper Significance

- This paper first showed the experimental benefit of CPM in the healing of articular cartilage injuries and serves as the basis for recommending its clinical use.

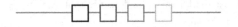

FEATURED ARTICLE

Authors: Horas U, Pelinkovic D, Herr G, Aigner T, Schnettler R.

Title: Autologous chondrocyte implantation and osteochondral cylinder transplantation in cartilage repair of the knee joint. A prospective, comparative trial.

Journal Information: *J Bone Joint Surg Am.* 2003;85:185–192.

A Top 100 Cited Articles in Clinical Orthopedic Sports Medicine

Study Design: Prospective Randomized Study

▶ Prospective randomized study of patients with femoral condyle articular cartilage lesions

  ▷ Transplantations of an autologous osteochondral cylinder graft (20 patients)

   » Transplant harvested from anterior superior aspect of the condyle

   » In 7 cases this harvest was not adequate and additional graft was harvested from the posterior femoral condyle.

  ▷ Transplantation of autologous chondrocytes (20 patients)

▶ Mean age 33.4 years (18 to 44 years), 23 men, 17 women

▶ Mean lesion size 3.75 cm² (3.2 to 5.6 cm²)

▶ Described as 2-year outcomes, but specific follow-up duration not specified

▶ Outcome measurements:

  ▷ Lysholm score

  ▷ Meyers score

  ▷ Tegner activity score

▶ Biopsy from representative patients evaluated with:

  ▷ Histological staining

  ▷ Immunohistochemistry

  ▷ Scanning electron microscopy

Results

▶ 17/20 patients in both groups reported substantial symptom improvement.

▶ Lysholm score

  ▷ Recovery after autologous chondrocyte implantation (ACI) was significantly slower than after osteochondral cylinder transplantation at 6, 12, and 24 months.

▶ Meyers score and Tegner activity score

  ▷ No difference between the 2 groups 2 years after treatment

▶ Follow-up arthroscopic examination and biopsy

  ▷ Performed in 6 patients after ACI

   » All biopsies showed complete, mechanically stable resurfacing of the defect that mainly consisted of fibrocartilage with localized areas of hyaline-like regenerative cartilage seen close to the subchondral bone.

  ▷ Performed in 5 patients after osteochondral cylinder transplantation

   » All biopsies showed an unreactive hyaline cartilage transplant adjacent to the resident hyaline cartilage, although a gap remained at the cartilage interface.

Conclusions

▶ Both treatments resulted in a decrease in symptoms.

▶ Symptom improvement provided by the ACI lagged behind that provided by the osteochondral cylinder transplantation.

▶ Defects treated with ACI were primarily filled with fibrocartilage.

▶ Defects treated with osteochondral cylinder transplants retained their hyaline character, although there was a persistent interface between the transplant and the surrounding original cartilage.

▶ Although autologous osteochondral cylinder transplantation is limited by donor-site availability, the authors consider it to be an appropriate treatment for articular cartilage lesions.

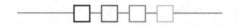

FEATURED ARTICLE

Authors: Bentley G, Biant LC, Carrington RW, Akmal M, Goldberg A, Williams AM, Skinner JA, Pringle J.

Title: A prospective, randomised comparison of autologous chondrocyte implantation versus mosaicplasty for osteochondral defects in the knee.

Journal Information: *J Bone Joint Surg Br.* 2003;85:223–230.

A Top 100 Cited Articles in Clinical Orthopedic Sports Medicine

---

Study Design: Prospective Randomized Study

▶ Prospective, randomized study of 100 patients with a symptomatic articular cartilage lesion of the knee

▷ Autologous chondrocyte implantation (58 patients)

» Mean 5.5 million cells (5 to 10 million) injected in second-stage procedure

» Used periosteum as covering membrane in 6 patients

» Used porcine collagen membrane (Chondro-Gide) in 46 cases (manuscript does not identify what was used for remaining 6 cases)

▷ Mosaicplasty (42 patients)

▶ Mean defect size 4.66 cm² (1 to 12.2 cm²)

- Defect location
  - ▷ 53 medial femoral condyle
  - ▷ 25 patella
  - ▷ 18 lateral femoral condyle
  - ▷ 3 trochlea
  - ▷ 1 lateral tibial plateau
- Mean symptom duration 7.2 years
- Mean age 31.3 years (16 to 49 years), 57 men, 43 women
- Mean follow-up 19 months (12 to 26 months)
- Outcome measurements
  - ▷ Cincinnati score
  - ▷ Stanmore score
  - ▷ Clinical assessment

Results

- Cincinnati and Stanmore scores (both identical)
  - ▷ Autologous chondrocyte implantation
    - » 88% excellent or good
  - ▷ Mosaicplasty
    - » 69% excellent or good
- Medial femoral condyle lesions (53 cases)
  - ▷ 88% excellent or good after ACI
  - ▷ 74% excellent or good after mosaicplasty ($P = 0.032$)
- Lateral femoral condyle lesions (18 cases)
  - ▷ 92% excellent or good after ACI
  - ▷ 40% excellent or good after mosaicplasty ($P = 0.182$)
- Patellar lesions (25 cases)
  - ▷ 85% excellent or good after ACI
  - ▷ 60% excellent or good after mosaicplasty ($P = 0.076$)
- Arthroscopic evaluation at 1 year
  - ▷ Autologous chondrocyte implantation (37 cases examined arthroscopically)
    - » 82% excellent or good (International Cartilage Repair Society grades of 1 or 2)
  - ▷ Mosaicplasty (23 cases examined arthroscopically)
    - » 34% excellent or good (International Cartilage Repair Society grades of 1 or 2)
    - » None of the 5 patients who underwent a mosaicplasty of a patellar lesion had a good arthroscopic result.

Conclusions

▶ Autologous chondrocyte implantation is superior to mosaicplasty for repair of knee articular defects.

▶ Autologous chondrocyte implantation is valuable for selected patients, providing healing of hyaline cartilage in chondral and osteochondral defects, dramatically reducing pain and disability.

▶ Use of Chondro-Gide porcine membrane as an alternative to periosteum was satisfactory, with no detectable difference in the healing.

▶ The authors concluded that the continued use of mosaicplasty was of dubious value.

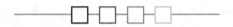

FEATURED ARTICLE

Authors: Bartlett W, Skinner JA, Gooding CR, Carrington RW, Flanagan AM, Briggs TW, Bentley G.

Title: Autologous chondrocyte implantation versus matrix-induced autologous chondrocyte implantation for osteochondral defects of the knee: a prospective, randomised study.

Journal Information: *J Bone Joint Surg Br.* 2005;87:640–645.

A Top 100 Cited Articles in Clinical Orthopedic Sports Medicine

---

Study Design: Prospective Randomized Study

▶ Prospective, randomized study of symptomatic chondral defects of the knee in 91 patients

  ▷ 44 treated with ACI using a porcine-derived type I/III collagen cover (ACI-C)

  ▷ 47 treated with matrix-induced autologous chondrocyte implantation (MACI) using a collagen bilayer seeded with chondrocytes

▶ The original ACI technique injected a suspension of cultured chondrocytes into a debrided chondral defect beneath a periosteal cover.

▶ Subsequently, a cover manufactured from porcine-derived type I/III collagen has been used.

▶ With both of these methods there is concern about uneven chondrocyte distribution within the defect and the potential for cell leakage.

▶ To overcome these problems, biodegradable scaffolds seeded with chondrocytes have been developed, such as the MACI technique.

▶ Mean age 33.5 years (15 to 49 years), 54 men, 37 women

▶ Mean lesion size 6.0 cm² (1.5 to 16 cm²)

▶ Lesion location (some knees had multiple lesion locations)

  ▷ 50 medial femoral condyle

  ▷ 11 lateral femoral condyle

  ▷ 36 patella

  ▷ 15 trochlea

▶ Outcome measurements

  ▷ Modified Cincinnati knee score

  ▷ Stanmore functional rating score

  ▷ Visual analogue score (VAS)

Results

▶ Both treatments resulted in improvement of the clinical score after 1 year.

▶ No significant difference between the 2 groups in:

  ▷ Modified Cincinnati knee score

  ▷ VAS

  ▷ Stanmore functional score

▶ Mean modified Cincinnati knee score

  ▷ Autologous chondrocyte implantation using a porcine-derived type I/III collagen cover (ACI-C)

    » 41.4 preop

    » 74.1 at 1 year ($P = 0.01$)

  ▷ Matrix-induced autologous chondrocyte implantation

    » 44.5 preop

    » 64.1 at 1 year ($P = 0.002$)

  ▷ Mean increase greater in MACI group, but not statistically significant (17.5 vs 19.6, $P = 0.32$)

▶ Arthroscopic assessment at 1 year (International Cartilage Repair Society score)

  ▷ No significant difference between the 2 groups in the arthroscopic graft appearance and histological findings

  ▷ 79.2% good to excellent in ACI-C group (24 patients underwent arthroscopy)

  ▷ 66.6% good to excellent in MACI group (18 patients underwent arthroscopy)

▷ Biopsies at 1 year showed hyaline-like cartilage or hyaline-like cartilage with fibrocartilage.
  » 43.9% of ACI-C treatment group
  » 36.4% of MACI treatment group
▷ Graft hypertrophy
  » 9% (4/44) in ACI-C treatment group
  » 6% (93/47) in MACI treatment group
▸ Reoperations
▷ 9% in each group

Conclusions

▸ Clinical, arthroscopic, and histological outcomes are comparable for both ACI-C and MACI treatment.
▸ The authors indicate that although the MACI technique is attractive (MACI is quicker to perform than ACI), further long-term studies are required before the technique is widely adopted since little is known about the durability of the MACI group.

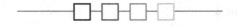

FEATURED ARTICLE

Authors: Knutsen G, Drogset JO, Engebretsen L, Grøntvedt T, Isaksen V, Ludvigsen TC, Roberts S, Solheim E, Strand T, Johansen O.

Title: A randomized trial comparing autologous chondrocyte implantation with microfracture. Findings at five years.

Journal Information: *J Bone Joint Surg Am.* 2007;89:2105–2112.

A Top 100 Cited Articles in Clinical Orthopedic Sports Medicine

---

Study Design: Prospective Randomized Study

▸ Randomized controlled trial of 80 patients without general osteoarthritis who had a single symptomatic cartilage defect on the femoral condyle in a stable knee

- Randomized to either
  - ▷ Autologous chondrocyte implantation (40 patients)
  - ▷ Microfracture (40 patients)
- Assessments
  - ▷ International Cartilage Repair Society Score
  - ▷ Lysholm score
  - ▷ SF-36
  - ▷ Tegner score
  - ▷ VAS for pain
- Follow-up exam performed by an independent observer at 1, 2, and 5 years
- Repeat arthroscopy with biopsy for histological evaluation was done at 2 years.

Results

- Both groups had significant clinical improvement compared to their preop condition at 2 and 5 years.
  - ▷ 72% of the patients had less pain.
  - ▷ 80% had improvement in the Lysholm score.
  - ▷ 72% had improvement in the SF-36 physical component score.
- Failures at 2 years
  - ▷ 2 in ACI group
  - ▷ 1 in microfracture group
- Failure at 5 years
  - ▷ 9 (23%) in ACI group
  - ▷ 9 (23%) in microfracture group
- Younger patients (< 30 years old) continued to do better in both groups ($P = 0.013$)
- No correlation between histological quality and clinical outcome
  - ▷ However, none of the patients with the best-quality cartilage (predominantly hyaline) at the 2-year mark had a later failure.
- 1/3 in each group had radiographic evidence of early osteoarthritis at 5 years

Conclusions

- Both methods provided satisfactory results in 77% of the patients at 5 years.
- No significant difference in the clinical and radiographic results between the 2 groups.
- No correlation between the histological findings and the clinical outcome.
- 1/3 of patients had early radiographic signs of osteoarthritis at 5 years.

▶ Authors stated that further long-term follow-up is needed to determine if one method is superior and to study the osteoarthritis progression.

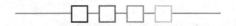

FEATURED ARTICLE

Authors: Steadman JR, Briggs KK, Rodrigo JJ, Kocher MS, Gill TJ, Rodkey WG.

Title: Outcomes of microfracture for traumatic chondral defects of the knee: average 11-year follow-up.

Journal Information: *Arthroscopy.* 2003;19:477–484.

A Top 100 Cited Articles in Clinical Orthopedic Sports Medicine

---

Study Design: Retrospective Review

▶ 72 patients (75 knees) treated arthroscopically with microfracture for full-thickness traumatic defects of the knee

▶ 95% (71 knees in 68 patients) were available for follow-up.

▶ Average age 30.4 years (13 to 45 years), 45 men, 23 women

▶ Average follow-up 11.3 years (7 to 17 years)

▶ Inclusion criteria

  ▷ Traumatic full-thickness chondral defect

  ▷ No meniscus or ligament injury

  ▷ Age ≤ 45 years

▶ Assessment

  ▷ Annual self-administered preop and post-op questionnaire

  ▷ Lysholm score

  ▷ Tegner score

  ▷ SF-36

  ▷ Western Ontario and McMaster Universities Arthritis Index (WOMAC)

Results

▶ Significant improvement in average Lysholm score ($P < 0.05$)

  ▷ 59 preop

▷ 89 at final follow-up

▶ Significant improvement in average Tegner score ($P < 0.05$)

▷ 3 preop

▷ Six at final follow-up

▶ 80% of patients rated themselves as "improved" at 7 years post-op.

▶ Treatment was considered a failure in 2 patients.

▶ Younger age was a predictor of functional improvement.

▷ Patients < 35 years had greater improvement in Lysholm scores than patients 35 to 45 years old ($P < 0.048$).

Conclusion

▶ Patients ≤ 45 years of age who underwent the microfracture for full-thickness chondral defects, without associated meniscus or ligament pathology, showed statistically significant long-term improvement in function and reduction in pain.

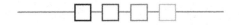

FEATURED ARTICLE

Authors: Peterson L, Minas T, Brittberg M, Lindahl A.

Title: Treatment of osteochondritis dissecans of the knee with autologous chondrocyte transplantation: results at two to ten years.

Journal Information: *J Bone Joint Surg Am.* 2003;85-A Suppl 2:17–24.

A Top 100 Cited Articles in Clinical Orthopedic Sports Medicine

---

Study Design: Cohort Study

▶ 58 patients with radiographically documented osteochondritis dissecans of the knee underwent treatment with autologous chondrocyte transplantation.

▶ 35 patients had juvenile-onset and 23 had adult-onset disease.

▶ 48 (83%) patients had undergone an average of 2.1 (0 to 8) prior operations.

▶ Mean duration of symptoms 7.8 years (0.1 to 36 years)

▶ Average age at time of treatment 26.4 years (14 to 52 years), 30 men, 28 women

- Mean lesion size 5.7 cm² (1.5 to 12.0 cm²), mean defect depth 7.8 mm (4 to 15 mm)
- Lesion location
  - 39 medial femoral condyle
  - 19 lateral femoral condyle
- Mean follow-up 5.6 years (1 to 10 years)
- Assessment
  - Modified Lysholm score
  - Modified Cincinnati (Noyes) knee score
  - Overall Cincinnati Knee Rating System
  - Wallgren-Tegner activity score
  - Overall Brittberg clinical grading score
  - Brittberg-Peterson functional assessment score
  - Questionnaire regarding the patient's perception of the surgical outcome
- 22 patients consented to arthroscopic second-look evaluation of graft integrity.

Results

- 91% had a good or excellent overall rating based on clinician evaluation.
- 93% had improvement on a patient self-assessment questionnaire.
  - Tegner-Wallgren, Lysholm, and Brittberg-Peterson VAS scores were all improved.
- Macroscopic quality of graft integrity averaged 11.2 on a 12-point scale, with only one graft having a score of < 9 points.
- 2 early post-op failures
- Only one patient who had a good or excellent rating at 2 years had a decline in clinical status at the latest follow-up.

Conclusions

- Treatment of osteochondritis dissecans knee lesions with autologous chondrocyte transplantation produces an integrated repair tissue with > 90% successful clinical results.
- The authors recommended wider use of autologous chondrocyte transplantation for treatment of osteochondritis dissecans of the knee.

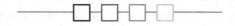

FEATURED ARTICLE

Authors: Peterson L, Vasiliadis H, Brittberg M, Lindahl A.

Title: Autologous chondrocyte implantation: a long-term follow-up.

Journal Information: *Am J Sports Med.* 2010;38:1117–1124.

Study Design: Prospective Cohort Study

▶ Study purpose: To investigate the long-term clinical results of ACI treated using a first-generation ACI technique and having a follow-up of 10 to 20 years

▶ In the first phase, autologous cartilage is harvested from a less weight-bearing area, usually the medial rim of the trochlea and occasionally from the lateral rim of the trochlea or femoral notch, and then cultured.

▶ In the second phase, cells are implanted into a debrided area of cartilage defect and a periosteal flap is harvested from the proximal medial tibia and sutured over the implant with the cambium layer facing the subchondral bone.

▶ Questionnaires sent to 341 patients

▷ Lysholm score

▷ Tegner-Wallgren score

▷ Brittberg-Peterson score

▷ Modified Cincinnati knee score

▷ Knee Injury and Osteoarthritis Outcome Score (KOOS) scores

▷ Patients also graded their status during the past 10 years as better, worse, or unchanged and were asked if they would do the operation again.

Results

▶ 66% (224/341) questionnaire response rate

▶ Mean cartilage lesion size was 5.3 cm^2.

▶ Mean time from ACI surgery 12.8 years (9.3 to 20.7 years)

▶ Average patient age at time of ACI 33.3 years (14 to 61 years)

▶ Average age at last follow-up evaluation 46 years (26 to 74 years)

▶ 74% (165/224) rated their status as better or the same as the previous years.

▶ 92% were satisfied and would have the ACI again.

▶ Average follow-up Lysholm, Tegner-Wallgren, and Brittberg-Peterson scores were all significantly improved compared to preop.

- Average Lysholm score
  - 60.3 preop
  - 69.5 at last follow-up ($P = 0.009$)
- Average Tegner-Wallgren score
  - 7.2 preop
  - 8.2 at last follow-up ($P = 0.002$)
- Average Brittberg-Peterson score
  - 59.4 preop
  - 40.9 at last follow-up ($P < 0.001$)
- KOOS at last follow-up
  - Average 74.8 for pain
  - Average 63 for symptoms
  - Average 81 for activities of daily living
  - Average 41.5 for sports
  - Average 49.3 for quality of life
- Average Modified Cincinnati knee score at last follow-up 5.4
- Patients with bipolar lesions (18 patients with patellofemoral bipolar lesions, 2 with medial compartment bipolar lesions, and 2 with lateral compartment bipolar lesions) had a worse final outcome than patients with multiple unipolar lesions.
- Associated meniscal injuries or history of bone marrow–stimulating procedures did not appear to affect final outcome.
- Age at the time of ACI and lesion size did not correlate with final outcome.

Conclusions

- Autologous chondrocyte implantation is an effective and durable solution for the treatment of large full-thickness cartilage and osteochondral lesions of the knee.
- This study suggests that the clinical and functional outcomes of ACI remain high even 10 to 20 years after implantation.

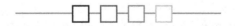

FEATURED ARTICLE

Authors: Meyers MH, Akeson W, Convery FR.

Title: Resurfacing the knee with fresh osteochondral allograft.

Journal Information: *J Bone Joint Surg Am.* 1989;71:704–713.

Study Design: Retrospective Review

▶ 58 consecutive patients (59 knees) treated with a fresh osteochondral allograft transplantation to the knee
▶ All patients had disabling pain after the failure of prior attempts to correct the problem surgically.
▶ 39 patients (40 knees) were available for follow-up at 2 to 10 years.
  ▷ 10 osteochondritis dissecans femoral condyle
  ▷ 3 trauma femoral condyle defects
  ▷ 3 avascular necrosis femoral condyle
  ▷ 5 chondromalacia patella
  ▷ 2 degenerative arthritis patella
  ▷ 7 traumatic arthritis tibial plateau
  ▷ 10 unicompartmental arthritis
▶ Osteochondral allografts were obtained from fresh cadavers of individuals aged 16 to 45 years old at time of death.
▶ Outcome measurements
  ▷ Merle d'Aubigné and Postel hip score
    ≫ 6 points maximum for pain, ambulatory status, and range of motion (ROM)
    ≫ 18 points = excellent
    ≫ 15 to 17 points = good
    ≫ 12 to 15 points = fair
    ≫ ≤ 12 points = poor
▶ Transplant considered successful if radiographs showed no evidence of degenerative arthritis; showed evidence of graft incorporation without collapse, narrowing of the joint space, or disintegration; and if the rating was excellent, good, or fair.
▶ Transplant considered a failure if the clinical rating was poor and there was radiographic evidence of absorption or collapse of the transplant or of narrowing of the joint space.

Results

- 22.5% (9/40) of transplants failed.
- 77.5% (31/40) were successful.
- Merle d'Aubigné and Postel hip score
  - ▷ 13/31 rated excellent
  - ▷ 14/31 rated good
  - ▷ 4/31 rated fair

Conclusions

- Fresh osteochondral allograft transplantation was a satisfactory intermediate procedure for the treatment of the disabling conditions, except for patients with unicompartmental traumatic arthritis.
- The authors recommend that a fresh osteochondral shell allograft transplantation be used for the treatment of:
  - ▷ Posttraumatic degenerative arthritis of the patella
  - ▷ Chondromalacia of the patellofemoral joint
  - ▷ Posttraumatic tibial plateau arthritis and traumatic defects
  - ▷ Traumatic defects, osteochondritis dissecans, and avascular necrosis of the femoral condyle
- The authors do not recommend the use of osteochondral allografts for unicompartmental degenerative knee arthritis that involves both the femur and tibia, since only 30% of such transplants were successful.
- The authors describe 8 criteria for successful osteochondral allograft transplantation.

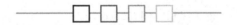

FEATURED ARTICLE

Authors: Levy YD, Görtz S, Pulido PA, McCauley JC, Bugbee WD.

Title: Do fresh osteochondral allografts successfully treat femoral condyle lesions?

Journal Information: *Clin Orthop Relat Res.* 2013;471:231–237.

Study Design: Retrospective Review

- ▶ Retrospective review of prospectively collected data on 122 patients (129 knees) who underwent fresh osteochondral allograft transplantation of the femoral condyle
- ▶ Mean age 32.8 years (15 to 68 years), 65 men, 57 women
- ▶ Mean graft size 8.1 cm² (1 to 27 cm²)
- ▶ Lesion location
  - ▷ 77 medial femoral condyle
  - ▷ 45 lateral femoral condyle
  - ▷ 7 both femoral condyles
- ▶ Outcome measurements
  - ▷ Modified Merle d'Aubigné-Postel (18 points)
  - ▷ International Knee Documentation Committee (IKDC)
  - ▷ Knee Society function (KS-F) scores
- ▶ Graft failure defined as revision osteochondral allografting or conversion to arthroplasty
- ▶ Minimum follow-up 2.4 years
  - ▷ Median follow-up 13.5 years
  - ▷ 91% (111/122) had more than 10 years of follow-up.

Results

- ▶ Mean modified Merle d'Aubigné-Postel score
  - ▷ 12.1 preop
  - ▷ 16 at follow-up (improved)
- ▶ Mean IKDC pain score
  - ▷ 7.0 preop
  - ▷ 3.8 at follow-up (improved)
- ▶ Mean IKDC function score
  - ▷ 3.4 preop
  - ▷ 7.2 at follow-up (improved)
- ▶ Mean Knee Society function score
  - ▷ 65.6 preop
  - ▷ 82.5 at follow-up (improved)
- ▶ 47% of knees (61/129) underwent reoperations.
- ▶ 24% of knees (31/129) failed at a mean of 7.2 years.
- ▶ Graft survivorship
  - ▷ 82% at 10 years
  - ▷ 74% at 15 years
  - ▷ 66% at 20 years

▸ Age > 30 years at time of surgery and having 2 or more prior knee surgeries were associated with allograft failure.

Conclusion

▸ Treatment of chondral and osteochondral femoral condyle lesions with fresh osteochondral allografts produces durable improvement in pain and function with 82% graft survivorship at 10 years.

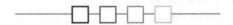

REVIEW PAPERS
Browne JE, Branch TP. Surgical alternatives for treatment of articular cartilage lesions. *J Am Acad Orthop Surg.* 2000;8:180–189.
Safran MR, Seiber K. The evidence for surgical repair of articular cartilage in the knee. *J Am Acad Orthop Surg.* 2010;18:259–266.
Sherman SL, Garrity J, Bauer K, Cook J, Stannard J, Bugbee W. Fresh osteochondral allograft transplantation for the knee: current concepts. *J Am Acad Orthop Surg.* 2014;22:121–133.

Anterior Cruciate Ligament Injury and Reconstruction

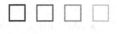

FEATURED ARTICLE

Authors: Bottoni CR, Liddell TR, Trainor TJ, Freccero DM, Lindell KK.

Title: Post-operative range of motion following anterior cruciate ligament reconstruction using autograft hamstrings: a prospective, randomized clinical trial of early versus delayed reconstructions.

Journal Information: *Am J Sports Med.* 2008;36:656–662.

2007 AAOSM O'Donoghue Award Winner

Study Design: Prospective Randomized Study

- 69 young athletic patients with an acute anterior cruciate ligament (ACL) tear
- Randomized to:
  - ▷ Early repair (within 21 days) 34 patients; mean time from injury to surgery 9 days (range 2 to 17 days)
  - ▷ Delayed repair (beyond 6 weeks) 35 patients; mean time from injury to surgery 85 days (range 42 to 192)
- Average age 27 years (range 18 to 43), 58 men, 11 women
- Identical surgical technique (autograft hamstring tendon) and post-op rehabilitation

▸ Articular cartilage and meniscal injuries were comparable between the 2 groups.
▸ Excluded patients with previous knee surgery and multiligamentous injuries
▸ Outcome assessments
  ▹ Range of motion
  ▹ KT-1000 arthrometer measurements
  ▹ Single assessment numeric evaluation (SANE)
  ▹ Lysholm score
  ▹ Tegner activity score

Results

▸ Average follow-up 366 days (range 185 to 869)
▸ No significant differences between the 2 treatment groups in:
  ▹ Degrees of extension or flexion loss
  ▹ Operative time
  ▹ KT-1000 arthrometer differences
  ▹ Subjective knee evaluations

Conclusion

▸ Early ACL reconstructions do not result in loss of motion or suboptimal clinical outcome as long as a rehabilitation protocol emphasizing extension and early range of motion is used.

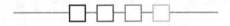

FEATURED ARTICLE

Authors: Marder RA, Raskind JR, Carroll M.

Title: Prospective evaluation of arthroscopically assisted anterior cruciate ligament reconstruction. Patellar tendon versus semitendinosus and gracilis tendons.

Journal Information: *Am J Sports Med*. 1991;19:478–484.

A Top 100 Cited Articles in Clinical Orthopedic Sports Medicine

Study Design: Prospective Randomized Study

▸ 80 consecutive patients with ACL tears underwent arthroscopically assisted reconstruction, alternating on a one-to-one basis with either.

  ▷ Autogenous patellar tendon

  ▷ Doubled semitendinosus and gracilis tendons

▸ No significant differences between the groups in age, sex, level of activity, and degree of laxity

▸ Standard post-op rehabilitation regimen was used for all patients

  ▷ Immediate passive knee extension

  ▷ Early stationary cycling

  ▷ Protected weight bearing for 6 weeks

  ▷ Avoidance of resisted terminal knee extension until 6 months

  ▷ Return to activity at 10 to 12 months post-op

▸ 8 patients had < 24 months follow-up and were excluded from analysis

▸ Average follow-up 29 months (24 to 40 months)

▸ Outcome assessments

  ▷ Zarins-Rowe subjective rating scale

  ▷ Lachman test

  ▷ Pivot shift test performed in external rotation

  ▷ Range of motion

  ▷ Circumferential thigh and calf measurements

  ▷ KT-1000 arthrometer measurement

  ▷ Isokinetic quadriceps and hamstring peak torque testing at 60 deg/sec using a Cybex dynamometer (20 patients from each group)

Results

▸ No significant differences between the two groups in:

  ▷ Subjective complaints (Zarins-Rowe subjective rating scale)

  ▷ Functional level

  ▷ KT-1000 measurements

▸ 24% (17/72) had anterior knee pain after ACL reconstruction.

▸ No difference between the groups in anterior knee pain

▸ 64% (46/72) returned to their preinjury level of activity.

▸ Mean KT-1000 scores

  ▷ 1.6 ± 1.4 mm in patellar tendon group

  ▷ 1.9 ± 1.3 mm in the semitendinosus and gracilis tendons group

▸ No statistically significant weakness in peak hamstring torque at 60 deg/sec in the group treated with double-looped semitendinosus and gracilis tendon

Conclusion

▸ Anterior cruciate ligament reconstruction performed with autogenous patellar tendon or combined semitendinosus and gracilis tendons results in comparable outcomes.

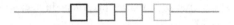

FEATURED ARTICLE

Authors: Hewett TE, Myer GD, Ford KR, Heidt RS Jr, Colosimo AJ, McLean SG, van den Bogert AJ, Paterno MV, Succop P.

Title: Biomechanical measures of neuromuscular control and valgus loading of the knee predict anterior cruciate ligament injury risk in female athletes: a prospective study.

Journal Information: *Am J Sports Med.* 2005;33:492–501.

A Top 100 Cited Articles in Clinical Orthopedic Sports Medicine

---

Study Design: Cohort Study

▸ 205 adolescent female athletes in the high-risk sports of soccer, basketball, and volleyball

▸ Prospectively measured for neuromuscular control during a jump-landing task

  ▷ Three-dimensional kinematics (joint angles)

  ▷ Joint loads using kinetics (joint moments)

▸ Analysis of variance, linear regression, and logistic regression were used to isolate predictors of risk for subsequent ACL rupture.

Results

▸ 9 athletes sustained an ACL rupture.

▸ They had significantly different knee posture and loading compared to the 196 who did not sustain an ACL rupture.

▸ Knee abduction angle at landing

  ▷ 8 degrees greater in ACL injured group ($P < 0.05$)

▸ Knee abduction moment

  ▷ 2.5 times greater in ACL injured group ($P < 0.001$)

- Ground reaction force
  - ▷ 20% higher in ACL injured group ($P < 0.05$)
- Stance time
  - ▷ 16% shorter in ACL injured group
- Increased motion, force, and moments occurred more quickly.
- Knee abduction moment predicted ACL injury status with 73% specificity and 78% sensitivity.
- Dynamic valgus measures showed a predictive r^2 of 0.88.

Conclusions

- Knee motion and knee loading during a landing task are predictors of ACL injury risk in female athletes.
- Female athletes with increased dynamic valgus and high abduction loads are at increased risk of ACL injury.
- Targeted interventions should be applied to this group to minimize the risk of ACL injury.

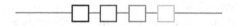

FEATURED ARTICLE

Authors: Beynnon BD, Uh BS, Johnson RJ, Abate JA, Nichols CE, Fleming BC, Poole AR, Roos H.

Title: Rehabilitation after anterior cruciate ligament reconstruction: a prospective, randomized, double-blind comparison of programs administered over 2 different time intervals.

Journal Information: *Am J Sports Med.* 2005;33:347–359.

2005 AAOSM O'Donoghue Award Winner

Study Design: Prospective Randomized Study

- 25 patients that underwent ACL reconstruction (bone–patellar tendon–bone graft) were randomized to:
  - ▷ Accelerated rehabilitation
  - ▷ Nonaccelerated rehabilitation
- Average age 32.7 (range 18 to 44 years), 11 men, 11 women

▶ 3 patients dropped out of study leaving 22 for analysis
  ▷ Accelerated rehab group—10 patients
  ▷ Nonaccelerated rehab group—12 patients

Rehabilitation Program

▶ Limits of knee range of motion, amount of weight bearing, and type of rehabilitation activity prescribed were common in the accelerated and nonaccelerated programs.
▶ However, these activities were incorporated over different time intervals.
  ▷ Accelerated program lasted 19 weeks
  ▷ Nonaccelerated program lasted 32 weeks
▶ Outcome assessments
  ▷ At time of surgery, 3, 6, 12, and 24 months post-op
  ▷ Clinical assessment
    » International Knee Documentation Committee (IKDC) assessment
    » Anterior posterior knee laxity, KT-1000 arthrometer measurement of joint laxity at 90 N and 130 N (primary outcome measure)
  ▷ Patient satisfaction
    » Self-administered Knee Osteoarthritis Outcome Score (KOOS)
  ▷ Functional performance
    » Single-legged hop test
  ▷ Cartilage metabolism (synovial fluid analysis)
    » Aggrecan turnover biomarker
    » Cleavage of type II collagen by collagenase
    » Synthesis of type II collagen

Results

▶ No difference in the increase of anterior knee laxity relative to baseline
  ▷ 2.2-mm increase relative to the normal knee in accelerated group
  ▷ 1.8-mm increase relative to the normal knee in nonaccelerated group
▶ The groups were similar in terms of clinical assessment, patient satisfaction, activity level, function, and response of the biomarkers.
▶ At 1 year post-op, synthesis of collagen and turnover of aggrecan remained elevated in both groups.

Conclusions

▶ Accelerated or nonaccelerated rehabilitation produces the same increase of anterior knee laxity following ACL reconstruction with a bone–patellar tendon–bone graft.

- ▸ Both rehabilitation programs resulted in similar clinical assessment, patient satisfaction, functional performance, and the biomarkers of articular cartilage metabolism.
- ▸ The authors expressed concern that the cartilage biomarkers remained elevated for an extended period.

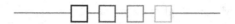

FEATURED ARTICLE

Authors: Fu FH, Shen W, Starman JS, Okeke N, Irrgang JJ.

Title: Primary anatomic double-bundle anterior cruciate ligament reconstruction: a preliminary 2-year prospective study.

Journal Information: *Am J Sports Med.* 2008;36:1263–1274.

Study Design: Cohort Study

- ▸ 100 consecutive patients who underwent anatomic double bundle (anteromedial and posterolateral) ACL reconstruction
- ▸ Average age 25.2 years (± 10.2 years), 62 women, 38 men
- ▸ Outcome measurements
  - ▷ Range of motion
  - ▷ Ligamentous laxity
  - ▷ Functional strength
  - ▷ IKDC Subjective Knee Form
  - ▷ Knee Outcome Survey (KOS)
  - ▷ SF-36
- ▸ 73 patients returned to clinic for follow-up exam
- ▸ Average follow-up 2.1 years

Results

- ▸ Side-to-side difference in range of motion was 2 degrees ± 3 degrees for extension and 2 degrees ± 5 degrees for flexion.

- Lachman test
  - ▷ 63% normal (< 3-mm side-to-side difference)
  - ▷ 33% "nearly" normal (3- to 5-mm side-to-side difference)
  - ▷ 2% abnormal (6- to 10-mm side-to-side difference)
- Pivot shift test
  - ▷ 94% normal
  - ▷ 6% "nearly" normal (glide but no clunk)
- Average KT-2000 arthrometer side-to-side measurements 1.0 mm ± 2.3 mm
- 8 graft failures
  - ▷ 7 had subsequent revision surgery.
- IKDC Subjective Knee Score = 85.0
- KOS Activities of Daily Living Score = 91.8
- Knee Outcome Survey Sports Activity Score = 87.0
- Outcome scores were similar to patients undergoing single-bundle ACL reconstruction.
- Self-described activity level
  - ▷ 51% normal
  - ▷ 35% nearly normal
- 72% of the subjects reported that they could participate in very strenuous or strenuous sports on a regular basis.

Conclusion

- Anatomic double-bundle ACL reconstruction results in good restoration of joint stability and patient-reported outcomes when evaluated 2 years after surgery.

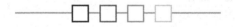

FEATURED ARTICLE

Authors: Freedman KB, D'Amato MJ, Nedeff DD, Kaz A, Bach BR Jr.

Title: Arthroscopic anterior cruciate ligament reconstruction: a meta-analysis comparing patellar tendon and hamstring tendon autografts.

Journal Information: *Am J Sports Med.* 2003;31:2–11.

A Top 100 Cited Articles in Clinical Orthopedic Sports Medicine

Study Design: Meta-analysis

▶ Meta-analysis of published studies that studied either patellar tendon allografts or hamstring tendon allografts in arthroscopic ACL reconstructions

▶ 34 studies met the inclusion criteria that included a minimum 2-year follow-up.

▶ 1,348 patients were treated with a patellar tendon autograft (21 studies).

▶ 628 patients were treated with a hamstring tendon autograft (13 studies).

▶ Mean age
  ▷ 25.9 years in patellar tendon group
  ▷ 25.4 years in hamstring tendon group

▶ Mean follow-up
  ▷ 46.3 months in patellar tendon group
  ▷ 34.2 months in hamstring tendon group

▶ Patellar tendon group had a significantly higher proportion of male patients ($P = 0.04$)
  ▷ Patellar tendon group 66.8% men
  ▷ Hamstring tendon group 62.1% men

Results

▶ Significantly lower rate of graft failure in the patellar tendon group
  ▷ 1.9% rate of graft failure in patellar tendon group
  ▷ 4.9% rate of graft failure in hamstring tendon group

▶ Significant higher proportion of patients in the patellar tendon group had a side-to-side difference of less than 3 mm on KT-1000 arthrometer testing
  ▷ 79% of patellar tendon group had < 3-mm side-to-side difference
  ▷ 73.8% of hamstring tendon group had < 3-mm side-to-side difference

▶ Higher rate of manipulation under anesthesia or lysis of adhesions in the patellar tendon group
  ▷ 6.3% rate in patellar tendon group
  ▷ 3.3% rate in hamstring tendon group

▶ Higher rate of anterior knee pain in the patellar tendon group
  ▷ 17.4% of patellar tendon group had anterior knee pain
  ▷ 11.5% of hamstring tendon group had anterior knee pain

▶ Higher incidence of hardware removal in the hamstring tendon group
  ▷ 5.5% of hamstring group underwent hardware removal
  ▷ 3.1% of patellar tendon group underwent hardware removal

Conclusions

▶ When undergoing ACL reconstruction, a patellar tendon autograft shows a modest advantage in providing better static knee stability, a lower rate of graft failure, and increased patient satisfaction, compared to a hamstring autograft.

▶ However, patients undergoing ACL reconstruction using a patellar tendon autograft had an increased rate of anterior knee pain and a higher rate of motion problems requiring surgical treatment.

▶ Both graft sources provided excellent return of function and a high rate of success.

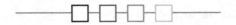

FEATURED ARTICLE

Author: Jones KG.

Title: Reconstruction of the anterior cruciate ligament: a technique using the central one-third of the patellar ligament.

Journal Information: *J Bone Joint Surg Am*. 1963;45:925–932.

A Top 100 Cited Articles in Clinical Orthopedic Sports Medicine

---

Study Design: Retrospective Review

▶ First reported description of using a central third patellar tendon autograft for ACL reconstruction

▶ Reports on 11 ACL reconstructions using a central third patellar tendon autograft

▶ Average age 19 years (14 to 39 years)

▶ Average follow-up 121 weeks (3 months to 5 years)

Results

▶ Average range of motion at follow-up 0 to 135 degrees

▶ 2 patients had occasional pain.

▶ 1 patient had occasional swelling after unusually heavy activity.

▶ None regarded the knee as unstable.

▶ 5 patients had a slight anterior drawer sign with the knee flexed 90 degrees.

- ▸ In full extension, all knees were completely stable.
- ▸ No significant complications

Conclusions

- ▸ The relatively simple described surgical technique substantially improved the function of the 11 knees in which it was performed.
- ▸ The authors recommended that a more extensive application of this basic technique, or some modification, seems warranted.

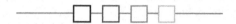

FEATURED ARTICLE

Authors: Shelbourne KD, Nitz P.

Title: Accelerated rehabilitation after anterior cruciate ligament reconstruction.

Journal Information: *Am J Sports Med.* 1990;18:292–299.

A Top 100 Cited Articles in Clinical Orthopedic Sports Medicine

---

Study Design: Retrospective Review

- ▸ Retrospective review of a prospectively collected database of subjective and objective outcomes following ACL reconstruction during 2 different time frames
  - ▷ 1984–1985 when patients were treated with a conventional post-op rehabilitation program
    - » Full weight bearing without brace was not permitted for 6 to 8 weeks.
    - » 138 patients, 90 men, 48 women
    - » 92% were followed throughout entire course of study
  - ▷ 1987–1988 when patients were treated with an accelerated post-op rehabilitation program
    - » 247 patients, 174 men, 73 women
    - » 98% were followed for varying lengths (12 to 30 months), 73 patients with > 2 year follow-up
- ▸ Accelerated rehabilitation program:
  - ▷ Full knee extension on the first post-op day.

▷ Immediate weight bearing according to the patient's tolerance.

▷ Patients with a 100-degree range of motion by the second post-op week participated in a guided exercise and strengthening program.

▷ Patients were permitted unlimited activities of daily living by the fourth post-op week.

▷ If the involved extremity Cybex strength scores were > 70% of the non-involved extremity at 8 weeks post-op, patients were allowed to return to light sports activities.

▷ Designed to overcome complications after ACL reconstruction (prolonged knee stiffness, limitation of complete extension, delay in strength recovery, anterior knee pain)

Results

▶ Quadriceps strength (% of uninvolved side)

  ▷ 4 to 6 months

    » 64% in conventional rehabilitation group

    » 75% in accelerated rehabilitation group ($P < 0.01$)

  ▷ 7 to 10 months

    » 75% in conventional rehabilitation group

    » 83% in accelerated rehabilitation group ($P < 0.01$)

  ▷ 1 year

    » 79% in conventional rehabilitation group

    » 91% in accelerated rehabilitation group

  ▷ > 1 year

    » 90% in conventional rehabilitation group

    » 92% in accelerated rehabilitation group

▶ Average range of motion

  ▷ 2 to 3 weeks

    » 5 to 75 degrees in conventional rehabilitation group

    » −4 to 104 degrees in accelerated rehabilitation group ($P < 0.01$)

  ▷ 6 to 7 weeks

    » 3 to 93 degrees in conventional rehabilitation group

    » −3 to 121 degrees in accelerated rehabilitation group ($P < 0.01$)

  ▷ 2 to 3 months

    » 2 to 121 degrees in conventional rehabilitation group

    » −3 to 130 degrees in accelerated rehabilitation group ($P < 0.01$)

  ▷ 6 to 7 months

    » 0 to 132 degrees in conventional rehabilitation group

    » −3 to 135 degrees in accelerated rehabilitation group ($P < 0.05$)

  ▷ 11 to 12 months

    ≫ 0 to 136 degrees in conventional rehabilitation group

    ≫ −4 to 139 degrees in accelerated rehabilitation group

▸ Scar resection required to obtain full knee extension

  ▷ 12% of patients in standard rehabilitation group

  ▷ 4% of patients in accelerated rehabilitation group

Conclusions

▸ The accelerated rehabilitation program offers advantages over conventional rehabilitation programs in terms of patient compliance and satisfaction and graft viability.

▸ Patients in the accelerated program returned to normal function and athletic activities sooner than patients in the conventional rehabilitation program.

▸ Patients in the accelerated program had fewer patellofemoral joint symptoms and a lower number of procedures required to obtain full knee extension.

▸ Range of motion, strength, and function can be achieved by an accelerated rehabilitation program without compromising stability or putting the graft at risk.

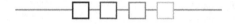

FEATURED ARTICLE

Authors: Desai N, Björnsson H, Musahl V, Bhandari M, Petzold M, Fu FH, Samuelsson K.

Title: Anatomic single- versus double-bundle ACL reconstruction: a meta-analysis.

Journal Information: *Knee Surg Sports Traumatol Arthrosc.* 2014;22:1009–1023.

Study Design: Meta-analysis

▸ Purpose: To compare effectiveness of anatomic double-bundle ACL reconstruction to anatomic single-bundle ACL reconstruction in restoring anterior-posterior laxity, rotatory laxity, and frequency of graft rupture.

- ▸ 15 studies with a total of 970 patients met their eligibility criteria.
  - ▹ 8 randomized controlled trials
  - ▹ 7 prospective cohort studies

Results

- ▸ Anatomic ACL double-bundle reconstruction demonstrated less anterior laxity.
  - ▹ Measured with KT-1000 arthrometer
    - » Standard mean difference = 0.36 (95% confidence interval 0.214 to 0.513, $P < 0.001$)
  - ▹ Measured with intra-operative computer navigation
    - » Standard mean difference = 0.29 (95% confidence interval 0.01 to 0.565, $P = 0.042$)
- ▸ Anatomic double-bundle ACL reconstruction compared to anatomic single-bundle ACL reconstruction did not lead to significant improvements in:
  - ▹ Pivot-shift test
  - ▹ Lachman test
  - ▹ Anterior drawer test
  - ▹ Total internal-external rotational laxity
  - ▹ Graft failure rates

Conclusions

- ▸ Anatomic double-bundle ACL reconstruction is superior to anatomic single-bundle reconstruction in terms of restoration of knee kinematics, primarily anterior-posterior laxity.
- ▸ It remains uncertain whether these improvements of laxity result in long-term improvement of clinical meaningful outcomes.

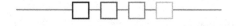

FEATURED ARTICLE

Authors: McDaniel WJ Jr, Dameron TB Jr.

Title: Untreated ruptures of the anterior cruciate ligament. A follow-up study.

Journal Information: *J Bone Joint Surg Am.* 1980;62:696–705.

A Top 100 Cited Articles in Clinical Orthopedic Sports Medicine

Study Design: Retrospective Review

▶ 50 patients (53 knees) with an ACL tear or attenuation (surgically verified at time of arthrotomy for treatment of a meniscal tear)

▶ Excluded patients with evidence of other ligamentous injuries

▶ Average age at injury 19.4 years (8 to 57 years), 42 men, 8 women

▶ Average time from injury to index arthrotomy 35 months

▶ Average follow-up 9.9 years from injury and 7 years from time of operation

▶ Average age at follow-up 29.3 years (12 to 66 years)

▶ Assessment

  ▷ Hospital for Special Surgery knee follow-up score (50-point scale based on interview and examination)

Results

▶ Hospital for Special Surgery knee follow-up score

  ▷ Average score 37.8

  ▷ 1 excellent (46 to 50 points)

  ▷ 10 good (41 to 45 points)

  ▷ 24 fair plus (36 to 40 points)

  ▷ 16 fair minus (31 to 35 points)

  ▷ 2 poor (26 to 30 points)

▶ Factors associated with better result:

  ▷ Regaining thigh circumference ≥ to normal side

  ▷ Stability to anterior and rotatory stresses

  ▷ Return to unrestricted sports activities

▶ Factors associated with a poorer result:

  ▷ Both medial and lateral meniscectomies

  ▷ Thigh atrophy

  ▷ Restriction of sports activities

  ▷ Instability to anterior and rotatory stresses

▶ 72% (38 patients) returned to strenuous sports.

▶ 47% (25 patients) reported no restriction due to the knee injury.

▶ Radiographic outcome (available for 49 patients, 52 knees)

  ▷ 13 knees had no radiographic abnormality.

  ▷ 28 knees had flattening or squaring of the femoral condyles.

  ▷ 8 knees had measureable medial joint-space narrowing.

  ▷ 3 knees had significant osteoarthritic changes.

▶ Thigh atrophy

  ▷ 24 patients had thigh atrophy on the injured side.

  ▷ 6 patients had thigh hypertrophy on the injured side.

- Range of motion
  - ▷ 18 patients had limited motion of the injured knee.
  - ▷ 6 patients had loss of flexion of 5 to 15 degrees
  - ▷ 12 patients had ≤5 degrees loss of full extension or of normal hyperextension.
- Instability
  - ▷ 10 knees had valgus instability up to 8 degrees with the knee in extension.
  - ▷ 29 knees had valgus instability up to 10 degrees with the knee flexed 30 degrees.
  - ▷ 3 knees had varus instability of 5 degrees with the knee in extension.
  - ▷ 8 knees had varus instability up to 8 degrees with the knee flexed 30 degrees.
  - ▷ 44 knees had a positive anterior drawer up to 2 cm with neutral tibial rotation.
  - ▷ 42 knees had a positive anterior drawer up to 2 cm with the tibia externally rotated.

Conclusions

- This study provides a baseline result for conservative treatment of ACL injuries and may be used for comparison in evaluating ACL repair procedures.
- The authors concluded, based on their analysis of 10 patients with articular cartilage degeneration noted at arthrotomy, that articular cartilage degenerative changes are more likely to be related to meniscal injuries and changes following meniscectomy than to ACL instability.
- The roentgenographic incidence of osteoarthritis at follow-up was low.
- Although there was a high incidence of anterior laxity, rotatory instability, and meniscal tears at follow-up, 72% of patients returned to strenuous sports and 47% reported no restrictions due to the knee injury.

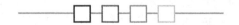

FEATURED ARTICLE

Authors: Corry IS, Webb JM, Clingeleffer AJ, Pinczewski LA.

Title: Arthroscopic reconstruction of the anterior cruciate ligament. A comparison of patellar tendon autograft and four-strand hamstring tendon autograft.

Journal Information: *Am J Sports Med.* 1999;27:444–454.

A Top 100 Cited Articles in Clinical Orthopedic Sports Medicine

Study Design: Cohort Comparison Study

▶ Compared 2 consecutive series of patients with isolated ACL injuries reconstructed with either:
  ▷ Patellar tendon autograft
  ▷ Hamstring tendon autograft
▶ All patients assessed prospectively
▶ First 90 patients reconstructed with a patellar tendon autograft
  ▷ 82 were available for 2-year follow-up.
▶ Next 90 patients reconstructed with a hamstring tendon autograft
  ▷ 85 were available for 2-year follow-up.
▶ Assessments
  ▷ Lysholm score
  ▷ IKDC scores
  ▷ Instrumented testing
  ▷ Thigh atrophy
  ▷ Kneeling pain

Results

▶ No difference between the groups in terms of ligament stability, range of motion, and general symptoms
▶ Median Lysholm knee score
  ▷ 95 in patellar tendon autograft group
  ▷ 95 in hamstring tendon autograft group
▶ IKDC scores
  ▷ Patellar tendon autograft group
    ≫ 48% normal
    ≫ 38% nearly normal

> » 9% abnormal
> » 5% severely abnormal
- ▶ Hamstring tendon autograft group
  > » 40% normal
  > » 53% nearly normal
  > » 5% abnormal
  > » 2% severely abnormal
- ▶ No difference in the return to level I or II sports, although more of the patellar tendon group reached level I
- ▶ KT-1000 arthrometer testing showed a slightly increased mean laxity in the female patients in the hamstring tendon graft group.
  - ▷ 2.5 mm (2.2 to 2.8 mm) in female hamstring autograft group
  - ▷ 1.0 mm (0.7 to 1.3 mm) in female patellar tendon autograft group
- ▶ Kneeling pain after reconstruction with the hamstring tendon autograft was significantly less common than with the patellar tendon autograft.
  - ▷ Anterior knee pain in patellar tendon autograft group
    > » 55% at 1 year, 31% at 2 years
  - ▷ Anterior knee pain in hamstring tendon autograft group
    > » 6% at 1 year, 6% at 2 years

Conclusions

- ▶ No difference in outcome of patients undergoing ACL reconstruction using patellar tendon vs hamstring autograft in terms of clinical stability, range of motion, general symptoms, and return to level I or II sports
- ▶ The lower rate of kneeling pain suggests lower donor-site morbidity with hamstring tendon harvest.

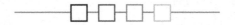

FEATURED ARTICLE

Authors: Noyes FR, Mooar PA, Matthews DS, Butler DL.

Title: The symptomatic anterior cruciate-deficient knee. Part I: The long-term functional disability in athletically active individuals

Journal Information: *J Bone Joint Surg Am.* 1983;65:154–162.

A Top 100 Cited Articles in Clinical Orthopedic Sports Medicine

Study Design: Retrospective Review

▶ 103 patients with symptomatic chronic laxity of the ACL without other associated major ligament deficiency or prior ligament reconstructive procedures.

▶ Study goal was to determine the long-term disability of patients whose knees demonstrated ACL laxity alone, without the superimposed variables of prior operative procedures or complicated by other types of ligament instability.

▶ 51 patients had undergone a meniscectomy, including 6 patients who had 2 meniscectomies.

▶ Average age 26 years (range 14.6 to 52.8 years), 75 men, 28 women

▶ 66% were past or present varsity athletes involved in high school or college sports.

▶ 33% participated in recreational sports only.

▶ Average 5.5 years after injury (range 3 months to 33.3 years)

▶ Patients divided into 2 groups:

▷ 64 patients who were < 5 years from injury (mean 2.2 years ± 1.4 years)

▷ 39 patients who were ≥ 5 years from injury (mean 11.2 years ± 6.8 years)

▶ Studies performed:

▷ 20-page questionnaire regarding original injury and treatment, subsequent injuries, participation in sports and routine activities, and symptoms

  » Symptoms of pain, swelling, and giving way were ranked as slight, moderate, or severe.

▷ Physical examination

▷ All included patients had an unequivocal anterior drawer sign, Lachman test, pivot-shift test, and flexion-rotation drawer test.

▷ Patients with medial or lateral laxity > 5 mm compared to other side were excluded.

Results

▶ In only 7/103 patients (6.8%) was the ACL tear diagnosis made by the original treating physician.

▶ 67 patients (65%) felt or heard a pop in the knee at the time of injury.

▶ Pain following original injury restricted normal activities > 3 weeks in 64/103 patients (62%)

▶ 85/103 patients (82%) returned to some form of sports activity after the original injury

▶ A significant reinjury occurred in:

▷ 36 patients (35%) within 6 months of the original injury

▷ 53 patients (51%) within 1 year of the original injury

▶ At follow-up, only 36 patients (35%) were participating in strenuous sports.

▶ A significant number of patients with longer follow-up had knee symptoms that affected their routine daily and recreational activities.

- Subjective moderate to severe overall disability reported in:
  - ▷ 32 patients (31%) for walking activities
  - ▷ 45 patients (44%) for overall routine activities of daily living
  - ▷ 77 patients (74%) for turning or twisting sports activities
- Pain
  - ▷ 31 patients (30%) reported pain during walking.
  - ▷ 48 patients (47%) reported pain during recreational activities.
  - ▷ 71 patients (71%) reported pain during strenuous sports activities.
- Instability
  - ▷ 22 patients (21%) reported giving way during walking.
  - ▷ 34 patients (33%) reported giving way during recreational activities.
  - ▷ 66 patients (65%) reported giving way during strenuous sport activities.
- Joint swelling occurred 4 to 5 times more often in patients who had the injury for the longest time (subset of 39 patients an average 11.2 years after injury).
- Statistically significant 2- to 4-fold increase in symptoms of pain and swelling related to activity in patients who had undergone a meniscectomy
- Radiographic evaluation
  - ▷ Radiographic arthritic changes related to the time after injury ($P < 0.01$)
  - ▷ Arthritic changes present in 17 patients (44%) in the subset of patients with the longest follow-up
  - ▷ Radiographic changes correlated statistically with participation in strenuous sports activities, with running activities, and with giving way.

Conclusions

- Significant functional disability occurs in patients with a symptomatic ACL-deficient knee.
- The degree of disability was related to length of time after the original injury.
- Initial disability occurs for sports activities.
- In the absence of treatment, reinjury is common, resulting in meniscal damage and subsequent joint arthritis.
- Later disability occurs for activities of daily living.

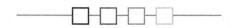

FEATURED ARTICLE

Authors: Noyes FR, Matthews DS, Mooar PA, Grood ES.

Title: The symptomatic anterior cruciate-deficient knee. Part II: The results of rehabilitation, activity-modification, and counseling on functional disability.

Journal Information: *J Bone Joint Surg.* 1983;65:163–174.

A Top 100 Cited Articles in Clinical Orthopedic Sports Medicine

---

Study Design: Retrospective Review

▶ Purpose:

  ▷ To analyze the results of a treatment program for chronic ACL-deficient knees that includes rehabilitation and activity modification

  ▷ To analyze factors that influence a patient's compliance with a rehabilitation program, including the extent that he or she understands the seriousness of the condition, his or her willingness to modify activities, and his or her willingness to follow an exercise program over many months

▶ 84 patients with symptoms of chronic ACL laxity were treated by a program designed to avoid recurrent symptoms.

  ▷ Rehabilitation

  ▷ Activity modification

  ▷ Knee brace for activities

  ▷ Periodic examination and follow-up to detect progressive joint deterioration

▶ Program failure was an indication for surgical reconstruction.

▶ Average age 28 years (range 17 to 54), 60 men, 24 women

▶ Original knee injury occurred an average of 8 years earlier

Eight-Point Treatment Program

▶ Identify and correct strength, power, and endurance deficits in all lower extremity muscle groups; rehabilitate for agility and neuromuscular coordination prior to sports participation

▶ Establish a weekly maintenance exercise program to prevent recurrence of muscle deficits

▶ Modification or substitution of specific types of activities or sports to eliminate or minimize jumping, cutting, and sudden turning or twisting that risk knee injury

▸ Counseling on future arthritis risk when activities are continued despite symptoms, particularly with chronic swelling or recurrent giving way that over time may cause joint deterioration

▸ Use of an appropriate knee brace for recreational and sports activities

▸ Assessment of functional knee disability after successful completion of the previous 5 steps (usually a minimum of 6 months are required to complete first 5 steps)

▸ Early use of arthroscopy for knees resistant to this program to define the true extent of joint deterioration for counseling purposes and potential treatment of meniscal or other problems that are preventing rehabilitation

▸ Periodic examination and follow-up to detect subtle joint deterioration before it is too late to modify activities and, when indicated, to recommend surgical treatment

Results

▸ Results were evaluated after 3 years by both subjective and objective criteria.

▸ 36 (30 patients) improved

▸ 32% (27 patients) no change

▸ 32% (27 patients) worsened, failed rehabilitation program

▸ 43% (36 patients) did not benefit from the program and were considered failures.

  ▷ 18 patients subsequently required reconstructive surgery because of such a functional disability.

  ▷ 18 additional patients became worse and were considering surgery.

▸ Frequency of knee reinjury was statistically correlated with chronic pain, swelling, and the overall severity of the knee condition.

▸ One third of the patients did not comply with recommended modifications or substitution of activities in order to prevent reinjury or recurrent symptoms.

Conclusions

▸ The 8-point treatment program was useful.

▸ It was difficult to predict initially which knees would or would not improve with the program, emphasizing the need for an initial nonoperative approach.

▸ Recurrent giving-way injuries, even if only 2 to 3 times a year may, over time, produce significant joint damage.

▸ Athletic activities resulting in even sporadic reinjury should be avoided, even when the symptoms between injuries are minimal.

▸ Individuals who continued active sports despite symptoms had an overall poor prognosis.

▶ The results of the study validate the usefulness of the 8-point treatment program, including the need for close follow-up, determining the individual patient's goals and demands, and activity modification and counseling.

▶ Arthroscopy is indicated in some knees to determine the extent of joint deterioration and, in some patients, the necessity for early surgical intervention.

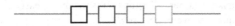

FEATURED ARTICLE

Authors: Daniel DM, Malcom LL, Losse G, Stone ML, Sachs R, Burks R.

Title: Instrumented measurement of anterior laxity of the knee.

Journal Information: *J Bone Joint Surg Am*. 1985;67:720–726.

A Top 100 Cited Articles in Clinical Orthopedic Sports Medicine

---

Study Design: Cohort Study

▶ Measured instrumented anterior-posterior knee laxity using a MEDMetric knee arthrometer (model KT-2000) in:

▷ 33 cadaver specimens

▷ 338 normal subjects

▷ 89 patients with unilateral ACL disruption

▶ Measured total anterior-posterior laxity produced by anterior and posterior loads of 89 N (20 pounds)

▶ Measured anterior compliance index

▶ Anterior compliance index = anterior displacement between an anterior load of 67 N and one of 89 N

Results

▶ Average anterior displacement at 89 N (20 pounds)

▷ 5.7 mm in normal subjects

▷ 13.0 mm in patients with an ACL disruption

▶ 92% of normal subjects had a left knee–right knee difference of ≤2 mm.

▶ 96% of patients with a unilateral ACL disruption had an injured knee–normal knee difference of >2 mm.

- 93% of normal subjects had a difference in the left-right compliance index of no more than 0.5 mm.
- 85% of patients with unilateral ACL disruption had a difference in the compliance index of the injured and normal sides of more than 0.5 mm.

Clinical Relevance and Conclusion

- Anterior cruciate ligament disruption results in increased anterior knee laxity that can be quantitatively measured.

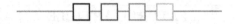

FEATURED ARTICLE

Authors: Daniel DM, Stone ML, Sachs R, Malcom L.

Title: Instrumented measurement of anterior knee laxity in patients with acute anterior cruciate ligament disruption.

Journal Information: *Am J Sports Med.* 1985;13:401–407.

Winner of the 1984 Clinical Studies Award
A Top 100 Cited Articles in Clinical Orthopedic Sports Medicine

---

Study Design: Cohort Study

- 138 patients studied within 2 weeks of injury that produced their first traumatic knee hemarthrosis
- MEDmetric arthrometer (model KT-1000) used to measure anterior/posterior knee laxity
- 75 patients underwent knee arthroscopy.
    - 87% had an ACL tear.
    - 41% had meniscus tears.
    - 33 had arthrometer laxity tests under anesthesia.
- 120 normal subjects were tested to establish normal anterior laxity values.
- 3 tests were used to evaluate anterior laxity.
    - Anterior displacement difference between a 15- and 20-pound force (compliance index)
    - Anterior displacement with a 20-pound force
    - Anterior displacement with a high manually applied force

Results

- Normal subjects
  - ▷ Wide range of laxity with a small right knee–left knee difference
  - ▷ 20-pound anterior displacement ranged from 3 to 13.5 mm.
  - ▷ Average right knee–left knee difference 0.8 mm
  - ▷ 80% had a right-left difference of less than 2 mm.
- 53 patients with arthroscopically confirmed complete ACL tears that had a preop clinic knee laxity measurement
  - ▷ 20-pound anterior displacement difference between knees
    - » 5 normal measurement (≤1.5 mm)
    - » 15 equivocal (2 to 2.5 mm)
    - » 33 abnormal (≥3 mm)
- Anterior laxity indicative of ACL disruption in the acutely injured knee
  - ▷ 20-pound anterior drawer
    - » 10 to 13.5 mm = equivocal
    - » ≥14 mm = diagnostic for ACL disruption
  - ▷ Manual maximum anterior drawer
    - » 12 to 15 mm = equivocal
    - » ≥15 mm = diagnostic for ACL disruption
  - ▷ Compliance index
    - » 2 to 2.5 mm = equivocal
    - » ≥3 mm =diagnostic for ACL disruption
- Suggested arthrometer measurements of anterior laxity
  - ▷ Displacement difference between knees of ≤.5 mm = normal anterior laxity
  - ▷ Displacement difference between knees 2 to 2.5 mm = equivocal
  - ▷ Displacement difference between knees ≥3 mm = abnormal

Conclusion

- ACL disruption results in an increase in anterior laxity that can be quantitatively measured.

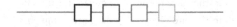

FEATURED ARTICLE

Authors: Daniel DM, Stone ML, Dobson BE, Fithian DC, Rossman DJ, Kaufman KR.

Title: Fate of the ACL-injured patient. A prospective outcome study.

Journal Information: *Am J Sports Med.* 1994;22:632–644.

1993 O'Donoghue Award Winner
A Top 100 Cited Articles in Clinical Orthopedic Sports Medicine

Study Design: Cohort Study

- 292 patients with an acute traumatic hemarthrosis
- 91% were 15 to 44 years old, 144 men, 88 women
- Average follow-up 64 months (46 to 113 months)
- KT-1000 arthrometer measurements within 90 days of injury showed that:
  - 56 knees were stable
  - 236 knees were unstable
    - 45 unstable knees underwent ACL reconstruction within 90 days of injury.
    - An additional forty-six patients underwent surgery that included ligament reconstruction > 90 days after injury.
- Joint arthrosis was documented by radiograph and bone scan.

Results

- 96% (144) of patients with an ACL disruption documented by arthroscopy had an injured knee minus normal knee displacement difference of ≥3 mm on KT-1000 arthrometer manual maximum test on their first examination.
- Early-phase (≤90 days after injury) arthroscopy in the 208 knees showed 51 medial meniscal tears and 71 lateral meniscal tears in 101 patients.
- 91 patients (31%) had ACL reconstructive surgery.
  - 45 patients in the early phase (≤90 days after injury)
  - 46 patients in the late phase (>90 days after injury)
- Factors that correlated with patients who had late surgery for a meniscal tear or an ACL reconstruction were:
  - Preinjury hours of sports participation
  - KT-1000 arthrometer measurements
  - Patient age (younger patients, correlated with hours of sports participation)

▶ Hours per year of sports participation and levels of sports participation decreased in all groups of patients.

▶ No patient changed occupation because of the knee injury.

▶ Reconstructed patients had a higher level of arthrosis by radiograph and bone scan.

Conclusions

▶ Instrumented measurement of anteroposterior knee displacement is a sensitive test for complete ACL disruption.

▶ There is a low probability (13%) that patients with an acute traumatic hemarthrosis that is found stable on instrumented examination will develop instability over the next 5 years.

▶ A high percentage (49%) of patients with an acute ACL injury have a meniscal tear, but not all patients with a torn meniscus need meniscal surgery.

▶ Total preinjury hours per year of levels I and II sport participation and displacement measurements were predictive of who would not require late surgery.

▶ Many ACL-injured patients who did not undergo knee reconstruction continued to participate in sports activities.

▶ Patients who had meniscal surgery had a greater incidence of joint arthrosis than those who did not have this surgery.

▶ Patients with an ACL injury who did not require meniscal surgery had a greater level of joint abnormalities by bone scan if they had ligament surgery than those who did not have ligament surgery.

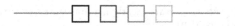

FEATURED ARTICLE

Author: The MARS Group.

Title: Effect of graft choice on the outcome of revision anterior cruciate ligament reconstruction in the Multicenter ACL Revision Study (MARS) cohort.

Journal Information: *Am J Sports Med.* 2014;42:2301–2310.

2014 AAOSM O'Donoghue Award Winner

Study Design: Cohort Study

- ▶ 1,205 patients (58% men) undergoing revision ACL reconstruction that were prospectively enrolled by 83 surgeons at 52 sites
- ▶ Median age 26 years
- ▶ Median time since last ACL reconstruction 3.4 years
- ▶ Autograft used for revision in 583 (48%) patients
- ▶ Allograft used for revision in 590 (49%) patients
- ▶ Both autograft and allograft used for revision in 32 (3%) patients
- ▶ Outcome measurements
  - ▷ IKDC
  - ▷ KOOS
  - ▷ Western Ontario and McMaster Universities Osteoarthritis Index (WOMAC)
  - ▷ Marx activity rating score
- ▶ Patients were followed up at 2 years.
- ▶ Multivariate regression used to determine the predictors (risk factors) of IKDC, KOOS, WOMAC, Marx scores, graft rerupture, and reoperation rate at 2 years following revision ACL surgery

Results

- ▶ Questionnaire follow-up was obtained for 989 subjects (82%).
- ▶ Telephone follow-up was obtained for 1112 (92%).
- ▶ IKDC, KOOS, and WOMAC scores (with the exception of the WOMAC stiffness subscale) all significantly improved at 2-year follow-up ($P < 0.001$).
- ▶ Marx activity score at 2 years was significant decreased from the initial score at enrollment ($P < 0.001$).
- ▶ Graft choice was a significant predictor of 2-year IKDC scores ($P = 0.017$).
- ▶ Use of an autograft for revision reconstruction predicted improved IKDC score ($P = 0.045$; odds ratio [OR] = 1.31; 95% CI, 1.01 to 1.70).
- ▶ Use of an autograft predicted an improved KOOS sports and recreation subscale score ($P = 0.037$; OR = 1.33; 95% CI, 1.02 to 1.73).
- ▶ Use of an autograft predicted improved KOOS quality-of-life subscale scores ($P = 0.031$; OR = 1.33; 95% CI, 1.03 to 1.73).
- ▶ Graft choice did not predict outcome scores for the KOOS symptoms and KOOS activities of daily living subscales.
- ▶ Graft choice was a significant predictor of 2-year Marx activity level scores ($P = 0.012$).
- ▶ Graft rerupture
  - ▷ Occurred in 37 of 1112 patients (3.3%) by the 2-year follow-up time
  - ▷ 24 allografts sustained a rerupture.

▷ 12 autografts sustained a rerupture.

▷ One combined allograft and autograft sustained a rerupture.

▷ Use of an autograft for revision resulted in patients being 2.78 times less likely to sustain a subsequent graft rupture compared to allograft ($P = 0.047$; 95% CI, 1.01 to 7.69).

Conclusions

▶ Use of autograft for revision ACL reconstruction results in improved sports function and patient-reported outcome measures.

▶ Use of an autograft shows a decreased risk in graft rerupture at 2-year follow-up.

▶ No differences were noted in rerupture or patient-reported outcomes between soft tissue and bone–patellar tendon–bone grafts.

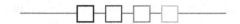

FEATURED ARTICLE

Authors: Sadoghi P, von Keudell A, Vavken P.

Title: Effectiveness of anterior cruciate ligament injury prevention training programs.

Journal Information: *J Bone Joint Surg Am.* 2012;94:769–776.

Study Design: Meta-analysis

▶ Study purpose

▷ To systematically review the literature on ACL injury prevention programs

▷ To perform a meta-analysis to address 3 questions

≫ What is the effectiveness of ACL injury prevention programs?

≫ Is there evidence for a "best" program?

≫ What is the quality of the current literature on ACL injury prevention?

Methods

▶ Conducted a systematic review using PubMed, MEDLINE, EMBASE, CINAHL (Cumulative Index to Nursing and Allied Health), and Cochrane Central Register of Controlled Trials databases

- Eight studies included in final analysis
- Extracted data on study design and clinical outcomes independently in triplicate
- Calculated pooled risk ratios and risk differences
- Risk difference used to estimate the number needed to treat (the number of individuals who would need to be treated to avoid one ACL tear)

Results

- Pooled risk ratio 0.38 (95% CI, 0.20 to 0.72), reflecting a significant reduction in the risk of ACL rupture in the prevention group ($P = 0.003$)
- Number needed to treat ranged from 5 to 187 in the individual studies.
- Pooled risk ratio stratified by sex
  ▷ Female athletes 0.48 (95% CI, 0.26 to 0.89)
  ▷ Male athletes 0.15 (95% CI, 0.08 to 0.28)
- Authors were unable to find conclusive evidence supporting any one specific type of intervention, but there was agreement among the studies that an ACL injury prevention program should include a minimum of 10 minutes of exercises 3 times per week that focus on neuromuscular training
- The scientific quality of the included studies was low, with only 2 studies having appropriate blinding and only 3 having adequate randomization.

Conclusions

- This study shows strong evidence to support a significant effect of ACL injury prevention programs.
- Pooled estimates suggest a substantial beneficial effect of ACL injury prevention programs.
- Anterior cruciate ligament injury prevention programs result in a 52% risk reduction in female athletes and 85% risk reduction in male athletes.

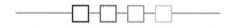

FEATURED ARTICLE

Authors: Gagnier JJ, Morgenstern H, Chess L.

Title: Interventions designed to prevent anterior cruciate ligament injuries in adolescents and adults: a systematic review and meta-analysis.

Journal Information: *Am J Sports Med.* 2013;41:1952–1962.

Study Design: Meta-analysis

▸ Study purpose: To examine the effect of neuromuscular and educational interventions on the incidence of ACL injuries through a systematic review and meta-analysis.

Methods

▸ MEDLINE, EMBASE, SPORTDiscus, CINAHL, the Cochrane Central Register of Controlled Trials, and Health Technology Assessment databases used to identify eligible studies

▸ Eligible studies assessed for risk of bias

▸ Meta-analyses performed on the estimated intervention effect using inverse-variance weighting, subgroup analysis, and random-effects meta-regression to estimate the overall (pooled) effect and explore heterogeneity of effect across studies

Results

▸ 8 cohort (observational) studies and 6 randomized trials were included in the analysis.

▸ These studies included approximately 27,000 participants.

▸ Random-effects meta-analysis yielded a pooled rate-ratio estimate of 0.485 (95% CI, 0.299 to 0.788; $P = 0.003$), indicating a lower ACL rate in the intervention groups.

▸ There was appreciable heterogeneity of the estimated effect across studies ($I^2 = 64\%$; $P = 0.001$).

▸ Estimated effect was stronger for studies that were not randomized, performed in the United States, conducted in soccer players, had a duration of follow-up > one season, had more hours of training per week in the intervention group, better compliance, and no dropouts

▹ Residual heterogeneity was still observed within subgroups of those variables ($I^2 > 50\%$; $P < 0.10$).

Conclusions

▸ Various types of neuromuscular and educational interventions appear to reduce the incidence rate of ACL injuries by approximately 50%.

▸ The estimated effect varied appreciably among studies and was not able to explain most of that variability.

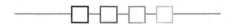

REVIEW ARTICLES

Frank JS, Gambacorta PL. Anterior cruciate ligament injuries in the skeletally immature athlete: diagnosis and management. *J Am Acad Orthop Surg*. 2013;21:78–87.

Fu FH, Bennet CH, Lattermann C, Ma CB. Current trends in anterior cruciate ligament reconstruction. Part 1: Biology and biomechanics of reconstruction. *Am J Sports Med*. 1999;27:821–830.

Murawski CD, van Eck CF, Irrgang JJ, Tashman S, Fu FH. Current concepts review: Operative treatment of primary anterior cruciate ligament rupture in adults. *J Bone Joint Surg Am*. 2014;96:685–694.

Prodromos CC, Fu FH, Howell SM, Johnson DH, Lawhorn K. Controversies in soft-tissue anterior cruciate ligament reconstruction: grafts, bundles, tunnels, fixation, and harvest. *J Am Acad Orthop Surg*. 2008;16:376–384.

Sutton KM, Bullock JM. Anterior cruciate ligament rupture: differences between males and females. *J Am Acad Orthop Surg*. 2013;21:41–50.

Posterior Cruciate Ligament Injury and Reconstruction

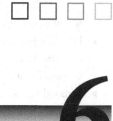

Chapter **6**

FEATURED ARTICLE

Authors: Tompkins M, Keller TC, Milewski MD, Gaskin CM, Brockmeier SF, Hart JM, Miller MD.

Title: Anatomic femoral tunnels in posterior cruciate ligament reconstruction: inside-out versus outside-in drilling.

Journal Information: *Am J Sports Med.* 2013;41:43–50.

Study Design: Cadaveric Study

▸ Purpose: To compare the ability of outside-in vs inside-out femoral tunnel drilling in placing the femoral tunnel aperture within the anatomic femoral footprint of the posterior cruciate ligament (PCL) and to evaluate the orientation of the tunnels within the medial femoral condyle

▸ 10 matched pairs of cadaver knees were randomized to either inside-out or outside-in femoral tunnel drilling.

▸ Computed tomography (CT) scans obtained before and after tunnel drilling to allow comparison of the PCL footprint to the drilled tunnel

▸ Measured % tunnel aperture contained within the native footprint and the distance from the center of the tunnel aperture to the center of the footprint

▸ Evaluated the orientation of the tunnels in the coronal and axial planes

Results

▸ % of tunnel placed within the native femoral footprint
  ▷ Outside-in technique 70.4% ± 23.7%

Miller MD, Mauffrey C, Hak DJ.
Rapid Reference Review in Sports Medicine:
Pivotal Papers Revealed (pp 99-104).
© 2016 Taylor & Francis Group.

▷ Inside-out technique 79.8% ± 16.7% ($P = 0.32$)
- Distance from center of femoral tunnel to center of native footprint
  ▷ Outside-in technique 4.9 ± 2.2 mm
  ▷ Inside-out technique 5.3 ± 2.0 mm ($P = 0.65$)
- Femoral tunnel angle in the coronal plane
  ▷ Outside-in technique 21.0 ± 9.9 degrees
  ▷ Inside-out technique 37.0 ± 10.3 degrees ($P = 0.002$)
- Femoral tunnel angle in the axial plane
  ▷ Outside-in technique 27.3 ± 4.8 degrees
  ▷ Inside-out technique 39.1 ± 11.5 degrees ($P = 0.01$)

Conclusions

- No difference between the outside-in and inside-out techniques to accurately place the femoral tunnel for PCL reconstruction within the PCL femoral footprint.
- The inside-out technique created femoral tunnels with a more vertical and anterior orientation than the outside-in technique.
- With the technique parameters used in this study, the inside-out technique produced gentler graft bends, which may affect graft strain and ultimately avoid graft failure.

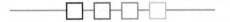

FEATURED ARTICLE

Authors: Clancy WG Jr, Shelbourne KD, Zoellner GB, Keene JS, Reider B, Rosenberg TD.

Title: Treatment of knee joint instability secondary to rupture of the posterior cruciate ligament. Report of a new procedure.

Journal Information: *J Bone Joint Surg Am*. 1983;65:310–322.

A Top 100 Cited Articles in Clinical Orthopedic Sports Medicine

Study Design: Cohort Study

- First reported description of using a central third patellar tendon autograft for PCL reconstruction
- Retrospective review of their initial experience in treating 48 patients using this technique
- 33 procedures performed for chronic instability

- 15 procedures performed for acute midsubstance PCL tears—these patients had intrasubstance repair of their PCL tear that was augmented by reconstruction with a central third patellar tendon autograft
- 48% of chronic cases had moderate to severe articular injury of the medial femoral condyle.
  - ▷ 71% of chronic cases that were from 2 to 4 years after injury showed articular damage.
  - ▷ 90% of chronic cases that were > 4 years after injury showed articular damage.
- Outcome grading
  - ▷ Excellent = full return to recreational or competitive sports or heavy manual labor with no or rare pain and no episodes of instability or effusions; absent or trace posterior drawer test
  - ▷ Good = full return to recreational or competitive sports or manual labor with only occasional pain with strenuous activities and none with activities of daily living and no episodes of instability or effusions; posterior drawer test ≤ 1+
  - ▷ Fair = significant but not disabling pain with sports or strenuous activities, but no or rare pain with the activities of daily living and no episodes of instability or effusions; posterior drawer test ≤ 1+
  - ▷ Failure = episodes of instability, persistent effusion, significant pain with normal activities; posterior drawer test ≥ 2+

Results

- 23/25 with a minimum 2-year follow-up returned for evaluation
  - ▷ 10 cases were performed for an acute repair and reconstruction.
    - » Average age 24 years (19 to 32 years), 9 men, 1 woman
    - » Average follow-up 41 months (30 to 57 months)
    - » All had a good or excellent result.
  - ▷ 13 cases were performed for chronic instability.
    - » Average age 25 years (19 to 35 years), 12 men, 1 woman
    - » Average follow-up 31 months (24 to 52 months)
    - » Operated on from 1 month to 20 years after original injury
    - » 11 had good or excellent results.

Conclusion

- Use of a central third patellar tendon for reconstruction in patients with acute midsubstance tears and patients with symptomatic chronic PCL instability is an effective procedure for achieving functional knee stability.

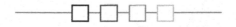

FEATURED ARTICLE

Authors: Del Buono A, Radmilovic J, Gargano G, Gatto S, Mafulli N.

Title: Augmentation or reconstruction of PCL? A quantitative review.

Journal Information: *Knee Surg Sports Traumatol Arthrosc.* 2013;21:1050–1063.

Study Design: Meta-analysis

- Purpose: To compare outcomes, advantages, and disadvantages of reconstructive vs augmentation procedures for treatment of PCL insufficiency, and to document the effectiveness and complications of surgery
- 24 studies met their inclusion criteria (used Coleman methodology score and Physiotherapy Evidence Database [scale])
  - 781 patients
    - Number of patients per studies ranged from 15 to 70.
  - 623 underwent PCL reconstruction
  - 158 underwent PCL augmentation
- Average modified Coleman methodology (a 10-criteria scoring list for methodological assessment of study quality) score 70.8 (60 to 82)

Results

- International Knee Documentation Committee (IKDC) assessment
  - Average rate of normal and nearly normal outcomes
    - 89.8% (85% to 93%) after PCL augmentation
    - 80.1% (57.2% to 100%) after PCL reconstruction
- Average Lysholm knee scores
  - 93.1 after PCL augmentation
  - 91 after double-bundle PCL reconstruction
  - 89 after single-bundle reconstruction
- KT-1000 difference
  - PCL augmentation
    - 8.8 mm average preop difference
    - 2.1 mm average post-op difference

▷ Posterior cruciate ligament reconstruction
  » 8.2 mm average preop difference
  » 2.3 mm average post-op difference
▶ Post-op Telos stress radiographic side-to-side difference
  ▷ Average 8.6 mm improvement after PCL augmentation
  ▷ Average 8.0 mm improvement after PCL reconstruction

Conclusions

▶ Augmentation and reconstruction procedures for PCL insufficiency are basically equivalent.
▶ More data are needed regarding long-term functional status, recovery to preinjury daily and sport activities, and occurrence of degenerative changes.

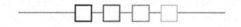

FEATURED ARTICLE

Authors: Yoon KH, Bae DK, Song SJ, Cho HJ, Lee JH.

Title: A prospective randomized study comparing arthroscopic single-bundle and double-bundle posterior cruciate ligament reconstructions preserving remnant fibers.

Journal Information: *Am J Sports Med.* 2011;39:474–480.

Study Design: Prospective Randomized Study

▶ 53 patents with PCL deficiency randomized to PCL reconstruction with an Achilles tendon allograft using the following technique:
  ▷ Double-bundle PCL reconstruction—28 cases
  ▷ Single-bundle PCL reconstruction—25 cases
▶ No statistically significant differences between the 2 groups in the mean age and interval between injury and operation
▶ Mean age 28 years, 45 men, 8 women
▶ Minimum 2-year follow-up
▶ Outcome measurements
  ▷ Preop and post-op range of motion
  ▷ Posterior stability by posterior stress radiography

▷ Tegner activity score

▷ Lysholm score

▷ IKDC subjective knee evaluation form

Results

▶ No difference in range of motion

▶ No difference in Tegner activity score

▶ No difference in Lysholm score

▶ No difference in IKDC subjective knee evaluation form

▶ Side-to-side difference in posterior translation significantly improved in both groups.

▶ No preop difference in posterior instability between the groups, but a significant difference at last follow-up.

▶ On the IKDC knee examination form, the double-bundle reconstruction group presented better results in grade distribution.

Conclusions

▶ The double-bundle reconstruction for PCL ruptures using the Achilles allograft showed better results in posterior stability and IKDC knee examination form compared to the single-bundle reconstruction.

▶ Although the difference of 1.4 mm in posterior stability was statistically significant, it is unclear that double-bundle reconstruction is definitely superior to single-bundle reconstruction clinically and functionally because there was no difference in the subjective scores.

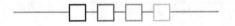

REVIEW ARTICLES

Fanelli GC, Beck JD, Edson CJ. Current concepts review: the posterior cruciate ligament. *J Knee Surg.* 2010;23:61–72.

Harner CD, Höher J. Current concepts: evaluation and management of posterior cruciate ligament injuries. *Am J Sports Med.* 1998;26:471–482.

Matava MJ, Ellis E, Gruber B. Surgical treatment of posterior cruciate ligament tears: an evolving technique. *J Am Acad Orthop* Surg. 2009;17:435–446.

Posterolateral Corner Injuries

Chapter 7

FEATURED ARTICLE

Authors: Stannard JP, Brown SL, Farris RC, McGwin G Jr, Volgas DA.

Title: The posterolateral corner of the knee: repair versus reconstruction.

Journal Information: *Am J Sports Med.* 2005;33:881–888.

Study Design: Cohort Study

▶ 56 patients with 57 posterolateral corner tears that had a minimum 2-year follow-up

  ▷ 35 treated by repair

    » 28 had multiligament knee injuries.

    » 7 had isolated posterolateral corner tears.

    » Criteria for repair included surgery within 3 weeks of injury and adequate tissue to support repair.

  ▷ 22 treated with reconstruction using the modified 2-tailed technique

    » 16 had multiligament knee injuries.

    » 6 had isolated posterolateral corner tears.

- ▶ 3 critical components of the deep layer of the posterolateral corner reconstructed using either a tibialis anterior or tibialis posterior allograft
  - ▷ Popliteus
  - ▷ Popliteofibular ligament
  - ▷ Lateral collateral ligament (LCL)
- ▶ Mean age 33 years (17 to 57 years), 35 men, 21 women
- ▶ Mean follow-up 33 months (24 to 59 months)
- ▶ Outcome measurements
  - ▷ Clinical knee examination
  - ▷ KT-2000 arthrometer measurements
  - ▷ Lysholm knee score
  - ▷ International Knee Documentation Committee (IKDC)
  - ▷ SF-36 scores
- ▶ Clinical examination included:
  - ▷ Varus instability tested at 0 and 30 degrees of flexion
  - ▷ Dial test conducted at both 30 and 90 degrees of flexion
  - ▷ 0 = < 5 degrees of difference between the 2 legs
  - ▷ 1+ = 5 to 10 degrees of difference
  - ▷ 2+ = 10 to 15 degrees of difference
  - ▷ 3+ = > 15 degrees of difference
  - ▷ Success = score of 0 or 1+
  - ▷ Failure = score of 2+ or 3+ on either the dial or varus stress test

Results

- ▶ Results clearly favored reconstruction over direct repair.
- ▶ Difference in success based on clinical exam stability between the repair and reconstruction groups was significant ($P = 0.03$)
  - ▷ Repair group (35 knees)
    - » 63% successful outcomes (22 knees)
    - » 37% failure (13 knees)
  - ▷ Reconstruction group (22 knees)
    - » 81% successful outcomes (20 knees)
    - » 9% failure (2 knees)
- ▶ Lysholm score
  - ▷ No difference in the final Lysholm scores
  - ▷ Mean 88.2 for successful repairs
  - ▷ Final mean 86.8 for failed repairs that were revised by reconstruction
  - ▷ Mean 89.6 for successful reconstructions
  - ▷ Final mean score 92 for failed posterolateral corner reconstructions that were revised

- ► Final IKDC objective scores
  - ▷ Mean score 60 at the most recent clinical evaluation
  - ▷ 26% (14) normal
  - ▷ 52% (28) near normal
  - ▷ 17% (9) abnormal
  - ▷ 6% (3) severely abnormal

Conclusion

- ► Reconstruction of posterolateral corner injuries using the 2-tailed technique resulted in superior results compared to treatment by repair.

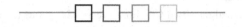

FEATURED ARTICLE
Authors: LaPrade RF, Johansen S, Agel J, Risberg MA, Moksnes H, Engebretsen L.
Title: Outcomes of an anatomic posterolateral knee reconstruction
Journal Information: *J Bone Joint Surg Am.* 2010;92:16–22.

Study Design: Cohort Study

- ► 64 patients with grade 3 chronic posterolateral instability
  - ▷ 2 centers (United States and Norway)
- ► 18 patients had an isolated posterolateral knee reconstruction.
- ► 46 patients underwent a single-stage multiple-ligament reconstruction that included reconstruction of one or both cruciate ligaments along with a posterolateral knee reconstruction.
- ► Average age 32 (18 to 58 years), 44 men, 20 women
- ► Average time from injury to reconstruction 4.4 years (2 months to 12 years)
- ► 54 (84%) were available for follow-up.
- ► Average follow-up 4.3 years (2 to 7.2 years)
- ► Assessments
  - ▷ Modified Cincinnati subjective score
  - ▷ IKDC subjective score

▷ IKDC objective score (completed preoperatively by the treating surgeon at one site and based on retrospective chart review at the other site and at the time of the follow-up examination at both sites)

▷ Grading based on findings of the individual physical examination pertinent to posterolateral knee instability

   » A = normal

   » B = nearly normal

   » C = abnormal

   » D = severely abnormal

Results

▶ Follow-up score

▷ Average total modified Cincinnati score 65.7 points (20 to 100 points)

▷ Average Cincinnati symptom subscore 32 points (8 to 50 points)

▷ Average Cincinnati function subscore 34 points (12 to 50 points)

▷ Average IKDC subjective score 62.6 points (20 to 100 points)

▷ No significant differences between the patients with isolated posterolateral knee reconstruction and those with multiple ligament reconstructions

▶ Significant improvement ($P < 0.001$) between the preop and post-op IKDC objective scores for:

▷ Varus opening at 20 degrees

▷ External rotation at 30 degrees

▷ Reverse pivot shift

▷ Single-leg hop

▶ Complications

▷ 1 post-op infection at 2 months requiring graft removal and revision posterolateral knee reconstruction

▷ 1 post-op common peroneal nerve neurapraxia that resolved by 4 weeks

▷ 3 recurrent posterolateral knee instability requiring revision posterolateral knee reconstruction

▷ 4 patients underwent removal of symptomatic hardware.

Conclusion

▶ Anatomic posterolateral reconstruction resulted in improved clinical outcomes and objective stability for patients with a grade 3 posterolateral knee injury.

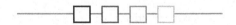

REVIEW ARTICLES

Ranawat A, Baker III CL, Henry S, Harner CD. Posterolateral corner injury of the knee: evaluation and management. *J Am Acad Orthop Surg.* 2008;16:506–518.

Veltri DM, Warren RF. Instructional course lecture: posterolateral instability of the knee. *J Bone Joint Surg.* 1994;76A:460–472.

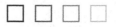

Medial Collateral Ligament Injuries

Chapter **8**

FEATURED ARTICLE

Author: Indelicato PA.

Title: Non-operative treatment of complete tears of the medial collateral ligament.

Journal Information: *J Bone Joint Surg Am.* 1983;65:323–329.

Study Design: Cohort Study

▸ Prospective cohort study of patients complete (grade III) isolated medial collateral ligament (MCL) tears

▸ All patients examined under anesthesia and arthroscopically (arthroscopic exam showed no structural damage to the anterior cruciate ligament [ACL-, menisci, or articular surfaces)

▸ Group 1: For 18 consecutive months all patients treated with primary surgical repair followed by 6 weeks of immobilization in a plaster cast and a well-defined, supervised rehabilitation program

▸ Group 2: For the next 18 months, all patients were treated without repair and immobilized of the knee in a plaster cast for 2 weeks, then in a cast-brace for 4 weeks, and the same well-defined, supervised rehabilitation program

▸ Mean age 19.4 years (17 to 38 years), 31 men, 5 women

▸ Group 1

  ▷ 16 patients

  ▷ Average follow-up 3.1 years

- Group 2
  - 20 patients
  - Average follow-up 2.4 years
- Objective scoring (up to 32 points awarded)
  - Assessed tenderness, effusion, soft tissue swelling, muscle weakness, loss of motion, ligament laxity
  - Anterior and posterior drawer signs
  - Valgus and varus stress testing with the knee in flexion and extension
    - Valgus stress test scoring
      - 5 points: Normal
      - 4 points: Mild instability (< 5 mm) with the knee in 30 degrees of flexion with a firm end point
      - 3 points: Moderate opening (5 to 10 mm) with the knee in 30 degrees of flexion, stability with the knee in extension, and a firm end point
      - 2 points: Instability (> 10 mm) with the knee in 30 degrees of flexion with a soft end point
      - 1 point: Gross medial instability without an end point
- Subjective scoring (up to 18 points for each item answered as "normal")
  - No pain or swelling
  - No difficulty with stair climbing or with cutting maneuvers
  - No loss of confidence in the knee
  - Functional abilities, including squatting, jumping, and duck walking were evaluated.
  - Ability to perform unrestricted athletic activity was graded
- Score grading
  - 41 to 50 points, good to excellent
  - 30 to 40 points, fair
  - > 30 points, poor

Results

- Group 1 (operative repair)
  - 15/16 patients good or excellent
- Group 2 (no repair)
  - 17/20 good or excellent
- Strength recovery measured by Cybex testing
  - Significantly faster in nonrepaired group that allowed accelerated rehabilitation ($P < 0.001$)
  - Group 1: 14.9 ± 1.5 weeks
  - Group 2: 11.3 ± 1.8 weeks

Conclusions

▸ Primary surgical repair of a complete (grade III) isolated MCL tear is not necessarily indicated.

▸ Rehabilitation was accelerated in patients treated in cast brace without primary repair.

▸ The key to success in treating grade III MCL injury is to establish that it is an isolated lesion with no associated damage to the ACL and menisci.

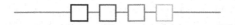

FEATURED ARTICLE
Authors: Woo SL-Y, Inoue M, McGurk-Burleson M, Gomez MA.
Title: Treatment of the medial collateral ligament injury. II: Structure and function of canine knees in response to differing treatment regimens.
Journal Information: *Am J Sports Med.* 1987;15:22–29.

Study Design: Animal Study

▸ Purpose: To evaluate the healing of the surgically transected canine MCL as a function of currently used clinical treatment regimens.

▸ The goal was to determine whether surgical repair with subsequent immobilization would result in more complete and rapid recovery than nonsurgical treatment without immobilization.

▸ 35 canine MCLs were surgically transected and treated using 3 clinically popular regimens.

  ▷ Group 1: No repair with cage and farm activities
   ≫ Animals sacrificed at 6, 12, and 48 weeks
  ▷ Group 2: Repair with 3 weeks immobilization
   ≫ Animals sacrificed at 6 and 12 weeks
  ▷ Group 3: Repair with 6 weeks immobilization
   ≫ Animals sacrificed at 6 and 12 weeks

▸ Assessments

  ▷ Quantitatively varus-valgus laxity of the knee joint
  ▷ Structural properties of the femur-MCL-tibia (FMT) complex

▷ Mechanical properties of the MCL substance at 6 and 12 weeks (also at 48 weeks for Group 1)

Results

▶ Group 1 animals had the best results.

   ▷ Varus-valgus laxity of the knee joint and the structural properties of the FMT complex returned to values comparable with the contralateral control by 12 weeks.

   ▷ Recovery of the mechanical properties of the MCL substance was slower and not complete even at 48 weeks.

▶ Prolonged immobilization was shown to have deleterious effects on MCL healing.

Conclusions

▶ The authors concluded that this study clearly demonstrated that conservative treatment with early mobilization, instead of surgical repair and prolonged immobilization, is the treatment of choice in the case of isolated MCL injury.

▶ The authors believe that conservative treatment is successful in the MCL-injured knee because valgus stability is maintained by the remaining joint structures, especially by the ACL.

▶ The authors recommend early motion once it is determined that the ACL is intact.

▶ This study also emphasized the importance and effectiveness of using various biomechanical parameters in addition to the conventional ultimate load to failure values to evaluate the progress of soft tissue repair.

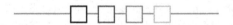

FEATURED ARTICLE

Authors: Woo SL-Y, Young EP, Ohland KJ, Marcin JP, Horibe S, Lin H-C.

Title: The effects of transection of the anterior cruciate ligament on healing of the medial collateral ligament: a biomechanical study of the knee in dogs.

Journal Information: *J Bone Joint Surg Am.* 1990;72:382–392.

Study Design: Animal Study

- Purpose: To examine the effects of partial and total loss of function of the ACL on healing of an unrepaired MCL injury
- 30 canines, sacrificed at 6 and 12 weeks
  - Group I: Isolated MCL transection
  - Group II: MCL transection and partial ACL transection
  - Group III: MCL transection and complete ACL transection
- Assessments
  - Quantitatively varus-valgus laxity of the knee joint
  - Structural properties of the FMT complex
  - Mechanical properties of the MCL substance at 6 and 12 weeks

Results

- Varus-valgus rotation of the knee
  - Largest in group III specimens at all time periods
  - 3.5 times greater than the control value at 12 weeks
  - Group I and group II specimens had large varus-valgus rotations at time zero, but these returned to the control values by 12 weeks.
- Structural properties of the FMT complex
  - Ultimate load for groups I and II reached the control values by 12 weeks
  - Ultimate load remained at 80% of controls in group III at 12 weeks
- Tensile strength at 6 weeks was markedly lower than control in all groups
- Tensile strength at 12 weeks
  - Group I: 52% of control
  - Group II: 45% of control
  - Group III: 14% of control
- All MCL injuries healed with a scar larger than the control ligament.
  - MCL cross-sectional area at 12 weeks
    - » Groups I and II: 2 times the control
    - » Group III: 5 times the control
- Articular surfaces
  - Group I: Normal
  - Group III: All showed grossly visible deterioration at 12 weeks along with marked periarticular osteophyte formation.

Conclusions

- Healing of transected MCL is adversely affected by concomitant ACL transection.
- Varus-valgus rotation and ligament mechanical properties failed to recover in knees that had combined ACL and transection.

▶ Structural properties of the FMT complex in tension recovered more rapidly due to the large mass of reparative tissue that formed in the MCL in animals with ACL deficiency.

▶ These findings suggest that the outcome after nonoperative management of combined MCL and ACL injuries may be less than ideal.

▶ The rapid return of the bone-ligament-bone structural properties may help explain the favorable functional outcomes reported in some clinical studies of combined ligamentous injuries, and the lack of agreement regarding patient outcomes may be due in part to differing methods of assessment.

▶ The poor quality of the healed ligamentous tissue and the articular degeneration seen in all cruciate-deficient knees in this study do not support nonoperative management with early mobilization in patients with combined MCL and ACL injuries.

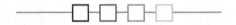

REVIEW ARTICLES

Miyamoto RG, Bosco JA, Sherman OH. Treatment of medial collateral ligament injuries. *J Am Acad Orthop Surg.* 2009;17:152–161.

Wijdicks CA, Griffith CJ, Johansen S, Engebretsen L, LaPrade RF. Current concepts review: injuries to the medial collateral ligament and associated medial structures of the knee. *J Bone Joint Surg Am.* 2010;92:1266–1280.

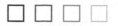

Lateral Collateral Ligament Injuries

Chapter **9**

FEATURED ARTICLE

Authors: Latimer HA, Tibone JE, ElAttrache NS, McMahon PJ.

Title: Reconstruction of the lateral collateral ligament of the knee with patellar tendon allograft: report of a new technique in combined ligament injuries.

Journal Information: *Am J Sports Med.* 1998;26:656–662.

Study Design: Retrospective Review

▸ 10 patients with posterolateral instability treated using a fresh-frozen bone–patellar tendon–bone allograft to reconstruct the lateral collateral ligament (LCL)

▸ Anatomic structures stabilizing the posterolateral corner of the knee are
  ▷ LCL
  ▷ Fabellofibular ligament
  ▷ Arcuate ligament

▸ All knees had from 1+ to 3+ varus instability and ≥20 degrees increased external rotation at 30 degrees of knee flexion preop.

▸ Cruciate ligaments were reconstructed with autograft or allograft

▸ Average age 32 years (19 to 40 years), 7 men, 3 women

▸ Average time from injury to surgery 19 months (3 to 45 months)

▸ Average follow-up 28 months (24 to 28 months)

▸ Fixation tunnels were placed in the fibular head and at the isometric point on the femur.

Miller MD, Mauffrey C, Hak DJ.
Rapid Reference Review in Sports Medicine:
Pivotal Papers Revealed (pp 117-121).
© 2016 Taylor & Francis Group.

▶ The fresh-frozen bone–patellar tendon–bone allograft was secured with interference screws.

Results

▶ Excessive external rotation at 30 degrees of flexion was corrected in 9/10 patients.
▶ Varus laxity at 30 degrees of flexion
  ▷ 6 patients had no varus laxity.
  ▷ 4 patients had 1+ varus laxity.
▶ Posterior drawer: 5 = 0, 5 = 1+
▶ Lachman test: 8 = 0, 2 = 1+
▶ Average Tegner score 4.6
▶ 5 patients returned to their preinjury level of activity.
▶ 4 patients returned to one level lower.

Conclusion

▶ The authors concluded that this was a promising new procedure for patients with instability resulting from lateral ligament injuries of the knee.

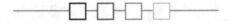

FEATURED ARTICLE

Authors: Ciccone WJ 2nd, Bratton DR, Weinstein DM, Walden DL, Elias JJ.

Title: Structural properties of lateral collateral ligament reconstruction at the fibular head.

Journal Information: *Am J Sports Med.* 2006;34:24–28.

Study Design: Cadaveric Study

▶ Purpose: To characterize the mechanical properties (especially the holding strength of the grafts within the fibular head) of LCL reconstruction using fibular interference fixation for soft tissue grafts with and without a bone plug.
▶ 10 intact cadaveric LCLs were tested to failure.

- ▶ Anatomic reconstruction of the LCL was performed by 2 different methods.
  - ▷ A socket for the interference screw was made in each fibular head with a 9-mm reamer.
  - ▷ 11 knees reconstructed with an Achilles allograft, including a calcaneal bone block—the bone block was secured to the fibula with a 9 × 23 mm interference screw.
  - ▷ 11 knees reconstructed with an Achilles allograft without a bone block—the ligament was secured to the fibula with a 9 × 23 mm interference screw.
- ▶ Reconstructed specimens were mechanically tested to failure with a force parallel to the fibular axis.

Results

- ▶ Intact specimens predominately failed through ligament rupture.
- ▶ Reconstructed ligaments consistently failed at the fibular head.
- ▶ Mean strength (± standard deviation)
  - ▷ Intact ligament 460 N (± 163 N)
  - ▷ Reconstruction with a bone plug 113 N (± 40 N)
  - ▷ Reconstruction without a bone plug 135 N (± 81 N)
- ▶ Mean stiffness (± standard deviation)
  - ▷ Intact ligament 82 N/mm (± 25 N/mm)
  - ▷ Reconstruction with a bone plug 36 N/mm (± 10 N/mm)
  - ▷ Reconstruction without a bone plug 34 N/mm (± 14 N/mm)
- ▶ Strength and stiffness were significantly ($P < 0.05$) greater for the intact ligaments than for either reconstruction group.
- ▶ Variation in strength was significantly larger for reconstruction without a bone plug than for reconstruction with a bone plug.

Conclusions

- ▶ The authors note that fibular interference fixation is increasingly being described, but this soft tissue fixation method should be used with care because of the inconsistency in the failure strength.
- ▶ Tension applied to LCLs reconstructed using fibular interference fixation should be limited immediately after surgery.

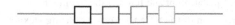

FEATURED ARTICLE

Authors: Meister BR, Michael SP, Moyer RA, Kelly JD, Schneck CD.

Title: Anatomy and kinematics of the lateral collateral ligament of the knee.

Journal Information: *Am J Sports Med*. 2000;28:869–878.

Study Design: Cadaveric Study

▸ The anatomy and kinematics of the LCL were studied in 10 unembalmed limbs and 20 isolated femurs and fibulas.

Results

▸ Average overall length of LCL 66 mm (59 to 74 mm) (Figure 9-1)

▸ Average greatest dimension of its thin middle portion was the anteroposterior dimension of 3.4 mm (3 to 4 mm)

▸ The center of the femoral attachment site was 3.7 mm posterior to the ridge of the lateral epicondyle, not at its apex.

▸ The authors identified a radiographic technique for operatively locating the anatomic femoral attachment site that is detailed in their manuscript.

▸ Kinematics of the LCL in neutral, internal, and external tibial rotation

  ▷ The ligament's orientation changes from an 11-degree posterior slope in extension to a 19-degree anterior slope in flexion.

  ▷ During knee flexion in neutral rotation, the distance between the femoral and fibular attachment sites of the LCL decreased to 88 percent of their value in full extension.

▸ Relaxation of the LCL with knee flexion has been widely reported and has traditionally been explained by the decreasing radius of curvature of the lateral femoral condyle and by the posterior position of the LCL relative to the knee flexion axis.

▸ This study's kinematic data suggest 2 other potentially contributing factors for relaxation of the LCL with knee flexion:

  ▷ Posterior translation of the femorotibial contact area

  ▷ Internal rotation of the tibia that occurs during flexion

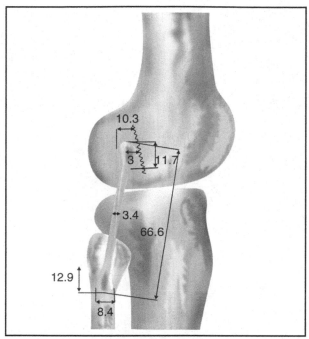

Figure 9-1. Average measurement data of the LCL femoral and fibular attachments.

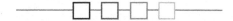

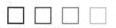

Knee Dislocations

Chapter 10

FEATURED ARTICLE

Authors: Stannard JP, Nuelle CW, McGwin G, Volgas DA.

Title: Hinged external fixation in the treatment of knee dislocations: a prospective randomized study.

Journal Information: *J Bone Joint Surg Am.* 2014;96:184–191.

Study Design: Prospective Randomized Study

▶ Patients with a knee dislocation that underwent ligament reconstruction randomized to:

  ▷ Use of a hinged knee brace following surgery (group A)

  ▷ Placement of a hinged external fixator (Compass Knee Hinge [Smith & Nephew]) for 6 weeks (group B)

▶ 100 patients with 103 knee dislocations enrolled

▶ 77 patients with 79 knee dislocations had a minimum 12-month follow-up

  ▷ 32 in hinged knee brace group

  ▷ 47 in hinged external fixator group

▶ Average age 35 years, 59 men, 18 women

▶ Mean follow-up 39 months (12 to 86 months)

▶ Assessments

  ▷ Physical examination

  ▷ Lysholm score

  ▷ International Knee Documentation Committee knee score

Miller MD, Mauffrey C, Hak DJ.
Rapid Reference Review in Sports Medicine:
Pivotal Papers Revealed (pp 123-128).
© 2016 Taylor & Francis Group.

▷ Visual analog scale pain score

▷ Status regarding return to work and activities

▶ Failure of reconstruction was defined as either 2+ or 3+ laxity on clinical exam, or for anterior cruciate ligament (ACL) and posterior cruciate ligament (PCL) reconstructions, a side-to-side difference of > 3 mm on KT-2000 arthrometer testing.

Results

▶ Failure of reconstruction

  ▷ Significant difference in ligament failure rate ($P < 0.001$; power > 0.8)

  ▷ Hinged knee brace group

    » 9 (29%) patients sustained a ligament failure.

    » 22 (21%) of 105 reconstructed individual ligaments failed.

  ▷ External fixator group

    » 7 (15%) patients sustained a ligament failure.

    » 11 (7%) of 157 reconstructed individual ligaments failed.

Conclusions

▶ Use of a hinged external fixator to supplement ligament reconstruction following knee dislocation was associated with fewer failed ligament reconstructions compared to use of a hinged knee brace.

▶ Use of a hinged external fixation should be considered to supplement initial reconstructive procedures in patients with highly unstable knee dislocations.

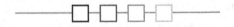

FEATURED ARTICLE

Authors: Barnes CJ, Pietrobon R, Higgins L.

Title: Does the pulse examination in patients with traumatic knee dislocation predict a surgical arterial injury? A meta-analysis.

Journal Information: *J Trauma.* 2002;53:1109–1114.

Study Design: Meta-analysis

▶ Purpose: To evaluate the diagnostic accuracy of pulse examination in detecting surgical arterial lesions associated with knee dislocation

- ▶ 7 articles met their study inclusion criteria.
- ▶ 284 knee dislocations and/or multiligamentous knee injuries

Results

- ▶ 52 knee injuries (18%) had associated arterial injury requiring surgery.
  - ▷ 45 presented with abnormal pedal pulses.
  - ▷ 7 presented with normal pedal pulses.
- ▶ 232 knee injuries (82%) did not have an arterial injury requiring surgery.
  - ▷ 211 presented with normal pedal pulses.
  - ▷ 21 presented with abnormal pedal pulses.
- ▶ Abnormal pedal pulses
  - ▷ Sensitivity 0.79 (95% confidence interval [CI], 0.64 to 0.89)
  - ▷ Specificity 0.91 (95% CI 0.78 to 0.96)
  - ▷ Positive predictive value 0.75 (95% CI, 0.61 to 0.83)
  - ▷ Negative predictive value 0.93 (95% CI, 0.85 to 0.96)

Conclusions

- ▶ Isolated presence of abnormal pedal pulses on initial examination of patients with knee dislocations is not sensitive enough to detect a surgical vascular injury.
- ▶ The authors recommend liberal use of angiography in patients with knee dislocations.
- ▶ The authors include an algorithm for the evaluation of patients sustaining a knee dislocation or an unstable knee due to multiligamentous injury.

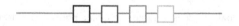

FEATURED ARTICLE
Authors: Mills WJ, Barei DP, McNair P.
Title: The value of the ankle-brachial index for diagnosing arterial injury after knee dislocation: a prospective study.
Journal Information: *J Trauma.* 2004;56:1261–1265.

Study Design: Cohort Study

- ▶ Prospective study of 38 patients sustaining a knee dislocation
- ▶ All patients underwent ankle-brachial index (ABI) after closed reduction.
  - ▷ To calculate ABI, the highest measured arterial pressure in the ankle or foot was divided by the higher of the brachial arterial pressures from both upper extremities.
  - ▷ Patients with an ABI < 0.90 underwent arteriography.
  - ▷ Patients with an ABI ≥ 0.90 were immobilized and admitted for serial examination and delayed arterial duplex evaluation.

Results

- ▶ 29% (11/38) of patients had an ABI < 0.90.
  - ▷ All 11 had an arterial injury requiring surgical treatment.
  - ▷ 2 patients had an expansile hematoma and underwent emergent exploration and revascularization with reverse saphenous vein grafting for a transected popliteal artery without undergoing preop arteriography.
  - ▷ 9 patients underwent emergent arteriography, which showed arterial injury requiring surgical intervention.
- ▶ 71% (27/38) of patients had an ABI ≥ 0.90.
  - ▷ None had vascular injury detectable by serial clinical examination or duplex ultrasonography.
- ▶ Sensitivity, specificity, and positive predictive value of an ABI < 0.90 was 100%.
- ▶ Negative predictive value of an ABI ≥ 0.90 was 100%.

Conclusions

- ▶ Ankle-brachial index is a rapid, reliable, noninvasive tool for diagnosing vascular injury associated with knee dislocation.
- ▶ Routine arteriography is not necessary for accurate diagnosis of a vascular injury.

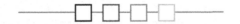

FEATURED ARTICLE

Authors: Stannard JP, Sheils TM, Lopez-Ben RR, McGwin G Jr, Robinson JT, Volgas DA.

Title: Vascular injuries in knee dislocations: the role of physical examination in determining the need for arteriography.

Journal Information: *J Bone Joint Surg Am.* 2004;86:910–915.

Study Design: Cohort Study

- Prospective outcome study of 130 consecutive patients (138 knees) who sustained an acute multiligamentous knee injury
- Vascular examination findings were used to determine need for arteriography.
- Patients with the following physical findings, consistent with a vascular injury, had arteriography:
  - Any decrease in pedal pulses, lower extremity color, or temperature
  - Expanding hematoma about the knee
  - History of an abnormal physical examination prior to presentation
- 4 patients (4 knees) lost to follow-up, leaving 126 patients (134 knees)
- Mean follow-up 19 months (8 to 48 months)

Results

- 9 patients (7%) had flow-limiting popliteal artery damage.
  - Knee dislocation classification according to the Wascher modification of the Schenck system
    - 1 knee dislocation-III (dislocations associated with tears of both cruciate ligaments and both posteromedial and posterolateral ligaments)
    - 7 knee dislocation-IV (dislocations associated with tears of both cruciate ligaments and both posteromedial and posterolateral ligaments)
    - 1 knee dislocation-V (dislocations associated with a periarticular fracture and multiple-ligament injuries)
- Prevalence of arterial damage associated with each dislocation classification
  - 0% for knee dislocation-I dislocation
  - 0% for knee dislocation-II dislocation
  - 2% for knee dislocation-III dislocation
  - 16% for knee dislocation-IV dislocation
  - 3% for knee dislocation-V dislocation

- 10 patients had abnormal physical examination findings.
  - ▷ 1 false-positive
  - ▷ 9 true-positive
- 17 patients had an arteriographic examination ordered by the attending orthopedic surgeon despite having normal physical examination findings, but none of these patients had angiographic findings that required vascular surgical treatment.
- There was a significant association between the findings on physical examination and a clinically important arterial injury ($P < 0.001$).
- Physical examination had a:
  - ▷ Positive predictive value of 90%
  - ▷ Negative predictive value of 100%
  - ▷ Sensitivity of 100%
  - ▷ Specificity of 99%

Conclusions

- Selective arteriography based on serial physical examinations is a safe and prudent policy after knee dislocation.
- There is a strong correlation between the physical examination results and the need for arteriography.
- Increased vigilance may be justified in the case of patients with knee dislocation-IV dislocation, which had the highest prevalence of vascular injury, for whom serial examinations should continue for at least 48 hours.

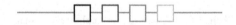

REVIEW ARTICLES

Levy BA, Fanelli GC, Whelan DB, et al. Controversies in the treatment of knee dislocations and multiligament reconstruction. *J Am Acad Orthop Surg*. 2009;17:197–206.

Rihn JA, Cha PS, Groff YJ, Harner CD. The acutely dislocated knee: evaluation and management. *J Am Acad Orthop Surg*. 2004;12:334–346.

Patellofemoral Disorders and Dislocations

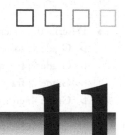

Chapter 11

CLASSIC ARTICLE
Author: Outerbridge RE.
Title: The etiology of chondromalacia patellae.
Journal Information: *J Bone Joint Surg Br.* 1961;43:752–757.

Study Design: Cohort Study

▶ The author carefully observed and recorded the condition of the patellar cartilage during 196 open meniscectomies.

▶ Noted a high frequency of chondromalacia patella, particularly after the age of 30

Results

▶ Abnormal patellar cartilage seen in 52% of cases
  ▷ Rate of abnormal cartilage by age group:
    » 50% in 24 patients < 20 years old
    » 35% in 48 patients 20 to 29 years old
    » 44% in 61 patients 30 to 39 years old
    » 71% in 42 patients 40 to 49 years old
    » 72% in 18 patients 50 to 59 years old
    » 67% in 3 patients 60 to 69 years old

▶ Found no relationship between the time or severity of injury and chondromalacia of patella

Miller MD, Mauffrey C, Hak DJ.
Rapid Reference Review in Sports Medicine:
Pivotal Papers Revealed (pp 129-137).
© 2016 Taylor & Francis Group.

- Described 4 macroscopic changes of cartilage:
  - ▷ Grade 1: softening and swelling of cartilage
  - ▷ Grade 2: fragmentation and fissuring in an area ≤ half inch in diameter
  - ▷ Grade 3: fragmentation and fissuring in an area > half inch in diameter
  - ▷ Grade 4: erosion of cartilage down to bone
- Reviewed 3 theories in the literature of the etiology of chondromalacia patellae:
  - ▷ Injury—the most common theory in the literature
  - ▷ Generalized constitutional tendency to cartilage degeneration
  - ▷ Patellofemoral contact with knee flexed > 90 degrees
  - ▷ The author felt that none of these theories adequately explained the etiology.
- Noted common site of origin on the medial patellar facet
- Described the anatomy of the medial femoral condyle, including the rim at its superior border, and the different anatomy at the upper border of the lateral femoral condyle
- Noted that the medial patellar facet is subjected to repeated pressure and shearing force during 15 to 30 degrees of flexion, and the part of the medial facet principally involved by this shearing force is the same area where the early changes of chondromalacia are seen
- Based on the anatomic findings, the author theorized that rubbing of the medial patellar facet on the rim at the upper border of the medial femoral condyle explains in part the etiology of chondromalacia patella.

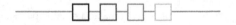

CLASSIC ARTICLE

Authors: Merchant AC, Mercer RL, Jacobsen RH, Cool CR.

Title: Roentgenographic analysis of patellofemoral congruence.

Journal Information: *J Bone Joint Surg Am.* 1974;56:1391–1396.

Study Design: Radiographic Review

- The authors describe a simple, accurate, and reproducible technique for obtaining axial radiographs of the patellofemoral joint ("sunrise" or "skyline" view).

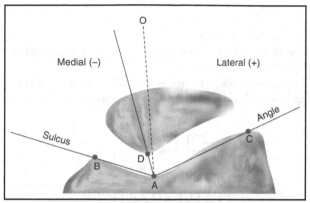

Figure 11-1. Identify the highest point of the medial (B) and lateral (C) condyles and the lowest point of the intercondylar sulcus (A). Bisect the sulcus angle (BAC) to establish the zero reference line (AO). Identify the lowest point on the articular ridge of the patella (D) and draw a line from A to D. The angle DAO is the congruence angle. All values medial to the zero reference line AO are designated as negative and those lateral as positive.

- The patient is positioned supine and the knees are flexed 45 degrees over the end of the table and the legs are supported.
- The central x-ray beam is inclined downward 30 degrees from the horizontal to strike the film cassette (placed distal to the patellae) at a right angle.
- Defined the congruence angle to measure patellofemoral congruence (Figure 11-1)

Measurement of Congruence Angle

- Identify the highest point of the medial (B) and lateral (C) condyles and the lowest point of the intercondylar sulcus (A).
- The angle, BAC, is the sulcus angle.
- Bisect the sulcus angle to establish the zero reference line (AO).
- Identify the lowest point on the articular ridge of the patella (D).
- Draw a line AD and project in anteriorly
- The angle DAO is the congruence angle.
- All values medial to the zero reference line AO are designated as minus and those lateral as plus

Results

- ▶ Studied 100 normal subjects
  - ▷ Average congruence angle was –6 degrees (standard deviation of 11 degrees)
  - ▷ Congruence angle > 16 degrees (lateral subluxation of the patella) was found to be abnormal at the ninety-fifth percentile.

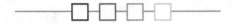

FEATURED ARTICLE

Authors: Hawkins RJ, Bell RH, Anisette G.

Title: Acute patellar dislocations. The natural history.

Journal Information: *Am J Sports Med.* 1986;14:117–120.

Study Design: Retrospective Review

- ▶ 27 patients sustaining primary patellar dislocations
- ▶ 20 were treated conservatively with immobilization and then physical therapy.
  - ▷ Average age 19 (13 to 39 years), 11 men, 9 women
  - ▷ Average follow-up 40 months (6 to 174 months)
  - ▷ 9 subsequently underwent arthroscopy.
- ▶ 7 underwent immediate open surgical stabilization and lateral release.
  - ▷ Average age 19 years (15 to 22 years), 3 men, 4 women
  - ▷ Average follow-up 27 months (19 to 52 months)

Results

- ▶ Instability
  - ▷ Conservative treatment group
    - ≫ 3 had a recurrent dislocation.
    - ≫ 4 had feelings of instability or "mistrust" of their knee, especially during activities involving external rotation and abduction.
  - ▷ Open treatment group
    - ≫ No recurrent dislocations
    - ≫ 2 had feelings of instability

- Pain and activity levels
  - ▷ Conservative treatment group
    - » 15 had pain of varying degrees.
    - » 6 had some limitation of activity.
  - ▷ Open treatment group
    - » 3 had pain of varying degrees.
    - » No activity limitation

Conclusions

- In the absence of predisposing factors, for patients sustaining a primary patellar dislocation, the authors recommend conservative treatment consisting of immobilization and physical therapy.
- In patients exhibiting a combination of predisposing signs (genu valgum, increased Q-angles, patella alta, or abnormal patellar configuration), primary surgical stabilization should be considered.
- In patients with no predisposing signs but with an osteochondral fragment, particularly one involving the articular surface, arthroscopy is useful to document its size and location and to treat by excision or reattachment.
- In patients with both predisposing signs and an osteochondral fragment, conservative treatment has a high risk for redislocation, and the authors recommend fragment excision with primary stabilization and realignment of the patellar mechanism.
- At least 30% to 50% of the patients sustaining a patellar dislocation will continue to have symptoms of instability and/or anterior knee pain, regardless of whether they are treated operatively or nonoperatively.

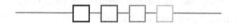

FEATURED ARTICLE

Authors: Insall J, Falvo KA, Wise DW.

Title: Chondromalacia patellae. A prospective study.

Journal Information: *J Bone Joint Surg Am.* 1976;58:1–8.

A Top 100 Cited Articles in Clinical Orthopedic Sports Medicine

Study Design: Cohort Study

▶ Prospective study of 105 arthrotomies for chondromalacia patellae

▶ 87 arthrotomies in 80 patients available for 2-year follow-up (range 2 to 5 years)

▶ Average age 22 years (13 to 61 years), 40 men, 40 women

▶ Patients were treated with either a proximal (53 knees) or distal (34 knees) patellar realignment procedure and either shaving or en bloc excision and drilling of the chondromalacic cartilage.

▶ A cylinder cast was applied for 6 weeks after distal realignment procedures, but no post-op immobilization was required after proximal realignment procedures.

Results

▶ Patella alta or an increased Q angle was found in most of the knees and was considered to be the usual cause of chondromalacia.

▶ Operative findings

  ▷ In 71% of cases, the lesion was located within an ellipse passing transversely across the central area of the patella, with sparing of the upper and lower third of the patellar articular surface.

  ▷ In 21% of cases, the lesion involved the medial facet alone.

  ▷ In 7% of cases, the lesion involved the lateral facet alone.

  ▷ Femoral changes were uncommon.

▶ Pain

  ▷ Constant aching pain was present preop in 84 knees.

  ▷ 35% (29 knees) had complete pain relief.

  ▷ 40% (34 knees) had partial but significant pain relief.

  ▷ 24% (20 knees) pain was unchanged

  ▷ 1 knee had increased pain.

▶ Complications

  ▷ 3 hematomas

  ▷ 5 knees required manipulation under anesthesia.

  ▷ No wound infections

  ▷ 7 knees required further surgery because of persistent or recurrent pain.

  ▷ Slight loss of flexion (10 to 15 degrees) was seen after distal realignment and occasionally after proximal realignment.

▶ Outcome

  ▷ Excellent: 13 knees (15%)

    » Complete relief of all preop symptoms, no abnormal objective findings on examination, and patients regarded the knee as "normal"

▷ Satisfactory: 53 knees (61%)
  » Some persistent discomfort or instability, subjective complaints of stiffness and swelling, clicking, retropatellar pain, or loss of motion, but patients regarded the knee as significantly improved
▷ Unchanged or worse: 21 knees (24%)
  » Unsatisfactory results usually because of failure to relieve pain

Conclusions

▶ Chondromalacia is usually a central lesion equally involving both medial and lateral patellar facets.
▶ Patellar realignment, together with excision of chondromalacic cartilage, gave a satisfactory result in 79% of cases.

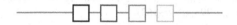

FEATURED ARTICLE

Authors: Petri M, Liodakis E, Hofmeister M, Despang FJ, Maier M, Balcarek P, Voigt C, Haasper C, Zeichen J, Stengel D, Krettek C, Frosch KH, Lill H, Jagodzinski M.

Title: Operative vs conservative treatment of traumatic patellar dislocation: results of a prospective randomized controlled clinical trial.

Journal Information: *Arch Orthop Trauma Surg.* 2013;133:209–213.

Study Design: Prospective Randomized Study

▶ Multicenter trial following first-time patellar dislocation randomized to:
  ▷ Conservative treatment
    » Knee brace with 0 to 60 degrees extension/flexion and partial weight bearing for the first 3 weeks
    » Motion advanced to 0 to 90 degrees extension/flexion and progression to full weight bearing for the following 3 weeks
  ▷ Operative treatment
    » Diagnostic arthroscopy followed by open medial soft tissue repairs with the option of performing a lateral release

- ▶ Inclusion criteria
    - ▷ Isolated, unilateral first-time traumatic patella dislocations
    - ▷ Ages 15 and 40 years
- ▶ Exclusion criteria
    - ▷ Recurrent dislocation
    - ▷ Significant anatomic deformities
    - ▷ Open injury
    - ▷ Pregnant or lactating patients
    - ▷ Osteochondral fragments requiring fixation
- ▶ 20 patients enrolled and randomized
- ▶ Average age 24.6 years (16 to 40 years), 13 men, 7 women
- ▶ Assessments at 6, 12, and 24 months
    - ▷ Kujala score (Kujala UM, et al. Scoring of patellofemoral disorders. *Arthroscopy*. 1993;9:159–163)
    - ▷ Any history of subsequent redislocation
    - ▷ Satisfaction

Results

- ▶ No significant difference between the treatment groups due to the small number of patients, but a tendency toward better results after operative treatment
- ▶ Mean Kujala score at 6 months
    - ▷ 78.6 in conservative treatment group
    - ▷ 80.3 in operative treatment group ($P = 0.842$)
- ▶ Mean Kujala score at 12 months
    - ▷ 79.9 in conservative treatment group
    - ▷ 88.9 in operative treatment group ($P = 0.165$)
- ▶ Mean Kujala score at 24 months
    - ▷ 81.3 in conservative treatment group
    - ▷ 87.5 in operative treatment group ($P = 0.339$)
- ▶ Redislocation rate at 24 months
    - ▷ 37.5% in conservative treatment group
    - ▷ 16.7% in operative treatment group ($P = 0.347$)

Conclusions

- ▶ No significant difference between conservative and operative treatment for patients after first-time traumatic patellar dislocation.
- ▶ Tendency toward a better Kujala score and lower redislocation rates for patients with operative treatment.

▸ The small number of patients is a limiting factor of the study, leading to results without statistical significance.

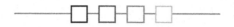

REVIEW ARTICLES

Bollier M, Fulkerson JP. The Role of Trochlear Dysplasia in Patellofemoral Instability. *J Am Acad Orthop Surg.* 2011;19:8–16.

Fukerson JP. Current concepts: diagnosis and treatment of patients with patellofemoral pain. *Am J Sports Med.* 2002;30:447–456.

Fulkerson JP. Patellofemoral pain disorders: evaluation and management. *J Am Acad Orthop Surg.* 1994;2:124–132.

Phillips CL, Silver DA, Schranz PJ, Mandalia V. The measurement of patellar height: a review of the methods of imaging. *J Bone Joint Surg Br.* 2010;92:1045–1053.

Post WR. Anterior knee pain: diagnosis and treatment. *J Am Acad Orthop Surg.* 2005;13:534–543.

Post WR. Current concepts: clinical evaluation of patients with patellofemoral disorders. *Arthroscopy.* 1999;15:841–851.

Redziniak DE, Diduch DR, Mihalko WM, et al. Instructional course lecture: Patellar instability. *J Bone Joint Surg Am.* 2009;91:2264–2275.

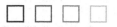

Miscellaneous Knee Topics

Chapter 12

FEATURED ARTICLE

Authors: Hewett TE, Lindenfeld TN, Riccobene JV, Noyes FR.

Title: The effect of neuromuscular training on the incidence of knee injury in female athletes. A prospective study.

Journal Information: *Am J Sports Med.* 1999;27:699–706.

A Top 100 Cited Articles in Clinical Orthopedic Sports Medicine

Study Design: Cohort Study

▶ Prospective study to evaluate the effect of neuromuscular training on the incidence of knee injury in female athletes

▶ Weekly monitoring of 2 groups of female athletes and 1 group of male athletes from 12 area high schools during each playing season (one school year or one season per sport)

  ▷ 15 teams of female athletes who underwent special training prior to sports participation (366 women)

    ≫ 6 weeks preseason neuromuscular training program that incorporated flexibility, plyometrics, and weight training to increase muscle strength and decrease landing forces

  ▷ 15 teams of female athletes who were not trained (463 women)

  ▷ 13 teams of male athletes who were not trained (434 men)

▶ Studied athletes participating in high school soccer, volleyball, and basketball because of the high level of jumping and cutting activity in these sports

▸ Weekly reports included the number of practice and competition exposures and mechanism of injury

Results

▸ 14 serious knee injuries in the 1263 athletes
  ▹ 2/366 trained female athletes sustained serious knee injuries (both were contact injuries)
  ▹ 10/463 untrained female athletes sustained serious knee injuries (8 were noncontact injuries)
  ▹ 2/434 male athletes sustained serious knee injuries (1 was a noncontact injury)
▸ Knee injury incidence per 1000 athlete-exposures
  ▹ 0.12 in trained female athletes
  ▹ 0.43 in untrained female athletes
  ▹ 0.09 in male athletes
▸ Untrained female athletes had 3.6 times higher incidence of knee injury than trained female athletes ($P = 0.05$).
▸ Untrained female athletes had 4.8 times higher incidence of knee injury than untrained male athletes ($P = 0.03$).
▸ Incidence of knee injury in trained female athletes was not significantly different from that in untrained male athletes ($P = 0.86$).
▸ Difference in the incidence of noncontact injuries between the female groups was significant ($P = 0.01$).

Conclusion

▸ This study demonstrated a decreased incidence of knee injury in female athletes after a specific plyometric training program.

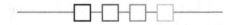

CLASSIC ARTICLE

Author: O'Donoghue DH.

Title: Surgical treatment of fresh injuries to the major ligaments of the knee.

Journal Information: *J Bone Joint Surg Am*. 1950;32:721–737.

Study Design: Retrospective Review

▶ Although subsequent authors have questioned the frequency of this injury pattern, this paper originally described a triad of injuries often referred to as the O'Donoghue triad.

▶ This injury is caused primarily by abduction and external rotation of the tibia on the femur, and the author has coined the term *the unhappy triad*.

▷ Medial collateral ligament (MCL) rupture

▷ Medial meniscus damage

▷ Anterior cruciate ligament (ACL) rupture

▶ Reports on the treatment of 22 patients with this injury triad

Results

▶ Emphasized the importance of physical examination at the time of injury to initiate timely surgical treatment

▷ Done before muscle spasm occurs

▷ Initial local shock may dull the pain.

▷ Swelling and hemarthrosis has not yet developed.

▶ Initial examination should include the following:

▷ Evaluate the degree of lateral instability, a valuable guide to the extent of MCL damage.

▷ Identify the exact area of tenderness, which serves to indicate the location of the tear or tears.

▷ Evaluate drawer sign, which documents the integrity of the ACL.

▷ Evaluate any restriction of extension, which when present early prior to muscle spasm is an almost infallible sign of meniscus damage.

Conclusions

▶ The author concluded that major improvement in the management of athletic injuries can be assured by early diagnosis and prompt definitive treatment.

▶ The author illustrates this concept through his review of the surgical management of patients sustaining an injury pattern that he coined *the unhappy triad*.

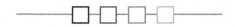

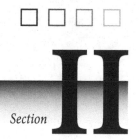

Section

II

Hip

Hip Labral Tears

FEATURED ARTICLE

Authors: Byrd JW, Jones KS.

Title: Primary repair of the acetabular labrum: outcomes with 2 years' follow-up.

Journal Information: *Arthroscopy.* 2014;30:588–592.

Study Design: Cohort Study

▶ Case series of 37 patients (38 hips) who underwent primary repair (using suture anchors) of a torn acetabular labrum and had a minimum 2-year follow-up

▶ Patients with pincer impingement undergoing labral mobilization for the purposes of acetabuloplasty were excluded.

▶ Assessment
  ▷ Modified Harris Hip Score

▶ Mean age 26 years (11 to 44 years), 26 women, 11 men

Results

▶ Outcome at 2 years
  ▷ 35 hips (92%) had good or excellent results.
  ▷ 35 hips (92%) showed improvement.
  ▷ 2 hips (6%) were unchanged.
  ▷ 1 hip (3%) had a poorer result.

- ▸ Mean modified Harris Hip Score
  - ▷ Preop 70.5 points
  - ▷ Post-op 89.4 points
- ▸ 4 patients underwent repeat arthroscopy at a mean of 10 months (5 to 15 months) post-op, and the labral repair site was found to be fully healed in each of these cases.
- ▸ No complications

Conclusion

- ▸ Primary repair of labral tears showed good clinical results with favorable outcomes and evidence of good healing.

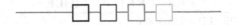

FEATURED ARTICLE
Authors: Byrd JW, Jones KS.
Title: Hip arthroscopy for labral pathology: prospective analysis with 10-year follow-up.
Journal Information: *Arthroscopy*. 2009;25:365–368.

Study Design: Cohort Study

- ▸ Case series of 29 patients (31 hips) who underwent arthroscopic treatment of an acetabular labral tear
- ▸ Labral lesions were treated by selective debridement of the damaged portion with creation of a stable transition zone to preserve healthy tissue.
- ▸ 3 patients died prior to their 10-year follow-up, leaving 26 patients for review.
- ▸ Average age 46 years (17 to 84 years), 13 men, 13 women
- ▸ Assessments
  - ▷ Modified Harris Hip Score preop and post-op at 3, 12, 24, 60, and 120 months

Results

- ▸ Median Harris Hip Score improvement was:
  - ▷ Preop 52 points
  - ▷ Post-op 81 points

- Patients with arthritis at the time of the index procedure did much poorer ($P < 0.001$)
  - ▷ 18 patients without preop arthritis
    - » 15 (83%) continued to show substantial improvement (≥ 18 points) at 10-year follow-up
  - ▷ 8 patients with associated preop arthritis
    - » 7 (88%) were converted to total hip arthroplasty at a mean of 63 months
- Patients with a history of a significant traumatic event fared much better (38 points) than those whose onset was insidious or even when a specific acute episode was identified; however, this difference was not statistically significant.
  - ▷ 4 traumatic injuries
    - » Preop Harris Hip Score 52, post-op 90
  - ▷ 13 insidious onset
    - » Preop Harris Hip Score 63, post-op 81
  - ▷ 9 patients with an acute episode (ie, twisting)
    - » Preop Harris Hip Score 43, post-op 31
- 2 patients underwent repeat arthroscopy, but still had a successful outcome at 10-year follow-up.
- No complications

Conclusions

- Selective debridement of symptomatic acetabular labral tears can result in favorable long-term results.
- Presence of arthritis at the time of the index procedure is a poor prognostic indicator, with uniformly poor results at 10 years.

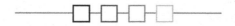

FEATURED ARTICLE

Authors: Dolan MM, Heyworth BE, Bedi A, Duke G, Kelly BT.

Title: CT reveals a high incidence of osseous abnormalities in hips with labral tears.

Journal Information: *Clin Orthop Relat Res.* 2010;469:831–838.

Study Design: Cohort Study

▶ There is a growing consensus that labral tears rarely occur in the absence of osseous abnormalities.

▶ Study purpose: To determine the presence of structural abnormalities in patients with acetabular labral tears using a standard computed tomography (CT) protocol.

Methods

▶ 135 consecutive patients with labral tears diagnosed by magnetic resonance imaging (MRI) with CT scans of the symptomatic hip were identified.

▶ CT scans were evaluated in a standard fashion to determine acetabular and femoral pathomorphologic features.

  ▷ Acetabular parameters measured

    ≫ Version

    ≫ Anterior center-edge angle

    ≫ Lateral center-edge angle

  ▷ Femoral parameters measured

    ≫ Version

    ≫ Alpha angle

    ≫ Neck-shaft angle

Results

▶ 90% (122/135) of hips had structural abnormalities.

▶ 76% (102/135) had an alpha angle > 50 degrees.

▶ 13% (18/135) had femoral version < 5 degrees.

▶ 16% (22/135) had femoral version > 25 degrees.

▶ 4% (5/135) had coxa valga.

- 43% (58/135) had acetabular retroversion.
  - ▷ 23/58 had isolated cranial retroversion.
  - ▷ 12/58 had isolated central retroversion.
  - ▷ 23/58 had combined cranial and central retroversion.
- 4% (5/135) had a lateral center-edge angle < 20 degrees.
- 55% (67/122) of hips with bony abnormalities had a combination of abnormalities.

Conclusions

- There is a very high incidence (90%) of structural abnormalities in patients with acetabular labral tears.
- This finding supports the concept that labral tears rarely occur in isolation.
- The presence of a labral tear should alert the physician to search for altered hip mechanics and underlying osseous pathomorphology.
- These structural abnormalities frequently occur in combination.
- Understanding the underlying morphologic features of the hip can help guide treatment.

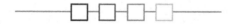

REVIEW ARTICLE

Safran MR. The acetabular labrum: anatomic and functional characteristics and rationale for surgical intervention. *J Am Acad Orthop Surg.* 2010;18:338–345.

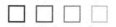

Femoroacetabular Impingement

Chapter 14

FEATURED ARTICLE

Authors: Beck M, Leunig, M, Parvizi J, Boutier V, Wyss D, Ganz R.

Title: Anterior femoroacetabular impingement; part II. Midterm results of surgical treatment.

Journal Information: *Clin Orthop.* 2004;418:67–73.

A Top 100 Cited Articles in Clinical Orthopedic Sports Medicine

---

Study Design: Cohort Study

▸ Review of prospectively collected data on 19 patients with femoroacetabular impingement (FAI) who underwent a surgical dislocation and treatment to improve the femoral neck offset

  ▷ Removal of any nonspherical portion of the femoral head

  ▷ Femoral offset creation by removal of the bony prominence on the anterolateral part of the head–neck junction

  ▷ Excision of the anterosuperior acetabular prominence when there was anterior overcover

  ▷ Resection of any fully degenerated or detached labrum

▸ Clinical and radiographic data collected prospectively with patients contacted at 2 months, 1 year, 2 years, 5 years, and every 3 years thereafter

▸ Average age 36 years (range 21 to 52 years), 14 men, 5 women

▸ Average follow-up 4.7 years (4 to 5.2 years)

Miller MD, Mauffrey C, Hak DJ.
*Rapid Reference Review in Sports Medicine:
Pivotal Papers Revealed (pp 151-162).*
© 2016 Taylor & Francis Group.

▶ Assessment
  ▷ Merle d'Aubigne and Postel hip score
    ≫ 6 points maximum for pain, ambulatory status, and range of motion (ROM)
    ≫ 17 to 18 points = very good to excellent
    ≫ 15 to 16 points = good
    ≫ 12 to 14 points = fair
    ≫ ≤11 points = poor

Results

▶ 13 excellent to good
▶ Pain score improved from 2.9 to 5.1 points at the last follow-up
▶ No femoral head avascular necrosis (AVN)
▶ 5 patients underwent subsequent total hip arthroplasty.
  ▷ 2 had grade 2 osteoarthrosis.
  ▷ 2 had grade 1 osteoarthrosis, but severe acetabular cartilage damage.
  ▷ 1 had untreated ossified labrum.
▶ There was no additional joint-space narrowing in the stable hips (hips with no femoral head subluxation into an acetabular cartilage defect).

Conclusions

▶ Surgical dislocation with correction of FAI yields good results in patients with early degenerative changes not exceeding grade 1.
▶ This procedure is not suitable for patients with advanced degenerative changes and extensive articular cartilage damage.

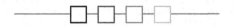

FEATURED ARTICLE

Authors: Ganz R, Parvizi J, Beck M, Leunig M, Nötzli H, Siebenrock KA.

Title: Femoroacetabular impingement a cause for osteoarthritis of the hip.

Journal Information: *Clin Orthop.* 2003;417:112–120.

A Top 100 Cited Articles in Clinical Orthopedic Sports Medicine

Classic Article

▶ In this article, the authors propose the theory that the development of early osteoarthritis for most nondysplastic hips is due to FAI.

▶ They base this theory on their clinical experience with more than 600 surgical dislocations of the hip that provided in situ inspection of the damage pattern and dynamic proof of its origin.

▶ The theory focuses more on motion than on axial loading of the hip.

▶ Distinct clinical, radiographic, and intraoperative parameters can be used to confirm the diagnosis of FAI.

▶ Surgical treatment centers on improving clearance for hip motion and alleviation of femoral abutment against the acetabular rim.

▶ The authors propose that early surgical intervention of FAI may decelerate the progression of the degenerative process.

▶ 2 distinct types of FAI can be distinguished based on the pattern and the various stages of chondral and labral injuries.

▶ Cam impingement
  ▷ Caused by jamming of an abnormal femoral head with increasing radius into the acetabulum during forceful motion, especially hip flexion
  ▷ Nonspherical portion of the femoral head abuts against the acetabular rim, leading to chondral abrasion and labral detachment.

▶ Pincer impingement
  ▷ Results from the linear contact between the acetabular rim and the femoral head–neck junction
  ▷ Femoral head may be morphologically normal and the abutment is due to acetabular abnormality such as coxa profunda or anterior overcoverage (acetabular retroversion)
  ▷ Continued impact of abutment results in labral degeneration with intrasubstance ganglion formation or rim ossification, which further deepens the acetabulum and worsens the overcoverage.
  ▷ The persistent anterior abutment with chronic leverage of the head in the acetabulum can result in chondral injury in the "contre-coup" region of the posteroinferior acetabulum.

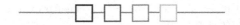

Study Design: Cohort Study

- Analysis of 26 hips with an isolated cam lesion who underwent surgical dislocation and treatment for FAI
  - Average age 32 years (21 to 51 years), 24 men, 2 women
- Analysis of 16 hips with an isolated pincer lesion who underwent surgical dislocation and treatment for FAI
  - Average age 40 years (24 to 57 years), 2 men, 14 women
- The authors treated a larger number of patients during this same time period, but more commonly the patients had combined deformities or had more advanced osteoarthritis and were excluded from this specific analysis.

Results

- The damage patterns in cam and pincer impingements differ considerably and require a different pathomechanical explanation.
- Cam impingement lesions (Figure 14–1A)
  - Absent anterior-to-anterolateral waisting of the junction of the femoral neck and head is the dominant feature.
  - In flexion, the eccentric part abuts the anterosuperior acetabulum and produces compression and shear stress at the junction between the labrum and cartilage and at the subchondral tidemark.
  - Causes damage to the anterosuperior acetabular cartilage with separation between the labrum and cartilage
  - During flexion the cartilage was sheared off by the nonspherical femoral head and the labrum remained undamaged.
- Pincer impingement lesions (Figure 14-1B)
  - A deep socket is the dominant feature, and hip ROM is limited by the overcovering acetabular rim.

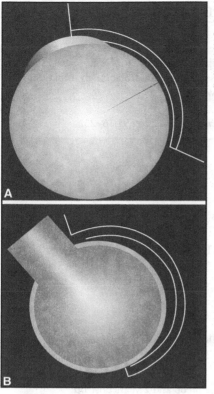

Figure 14-1. (A) Schematic representation of cam mechanism of femoroacetabular dysplasia where an abnormally shaped femoral head abuts on the acetabular rim. (B) Pincer mechanism where abutment is due to acetabular abnormality resulting in excessive acetabular coverage.

▷ At the limit of motion, the femoral neck abuts against the labrum, which acts like a bumper.

▷ Causes damage to the articular cartilage circumferentially but only involving a narrow strip

▷ During movement the labrum was crushed between the acetabular rim and the femoral neck, causing degeneration and ossification.

Conclusions

▶ The authors concluded that their study provides an explanation of the mechanism that is responsible for hip degeneration in patients with bony abnormalities, including pistol-grip deformity, tilt deformity, femoral anteversion, coxa profunda, coxa protrusion, and acetabular retroversion.

▶ Cam and pincer impingement are two basic mechanisms causing FAI, but they rarely occur in isolation.

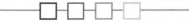

> **FEATURED ARTICLE**
>
> **Authors:** Philippon MJ, Briggs KK, Yen YM, Kuppersmith DA.
>
> **Title:** Outcomes following hip arthroscopy for femoroacetabu-
> lar impingement with associated chondrolabral dysfunction:
> minimum two-year follow-up.
>
> **Journal Information:** *J Bone Joint Surg Br.* 2009;91:16–23.

Study Design: Cohort Study

- Prospective review of 112 patients with FAI
- Inclusion criteria
  - ▷ Arthroscopic treatment for FAI and chondrolabral dysfunction
- Exclusion criteria
  - ▷ Bilateral hip arthroscopy
  - ▷ Avascular necrosis
  - ▷ Previous hip surgery
- Average age 40.6 years, 62 women, 50 men
- Average follow-up 2.3 years (2 to 2.9 years)
- Assessment
  - ▷ Self-administered questionnaire preop and 2 years post-op
  - ▷ Hip outcome score
  - ▷ Nonarthritic hip score
  - ▷ Modified Harris Hip Score (HHS)
  - ▷ Patient satisfaction with outcome (1 = unsatisfied, 10 = very satisfied)
- Surgical treatment
  - ▷ 23 patients underwent osteoplasty only for cam impingement.
  - ▷ 3 patients underwent rim trimming only for pincer impingement.
  - ▷ 86 patients underwent both procedures for mixed-type impingement.

Results

- Mean modified HHS
  - ▷ Preop 58
  - ▷ Follow-up 84
- Median follow-up patient satisfaction 9
- 10 patients underwent total hip replacement at a mean of 16 months (8 to 26 months) after arthroscopy.

- Predictors of a better outcome (multivariable analysis showed 3 independent predictors of the post-op modified HHS)
  ▷ Pre-op modified HHS score
  ▷ Joint-space narrowing ≥ 2 mm
  ▷ Repair of labral pathology instead of debridement

Conclusion

- Hip arthroscopy for FAI, accompanied by suitable rehabilitation, provides good short-term outcome and high patient satisfaction.

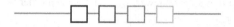

FEATURED ARTICLE

Authors: Agricola R, Heijboer MP, Ginai AZ, Roels P, Zadpoor AA, Verhaar JA, Weinans H, Waarsing JH.

Title: A cam deformity is gradually acquired during skeletal maturation in adolescent and young male soccer players: a prospective study with minimum 2-year follow-up.

Journal Information: *Am J Sports Med.* 2014;42:798–806.

Study Design: Cohort Study

- Purpose: To study whether a cam deformity can evolve over time in adolescents and examine whether clinical or radiographic features can predict the formation of a cam deformity.

Methods

- 63 preprofessional soccer players studied in Rotterdam, the Netherlands
- Average age 14.4 years (12 to 19 years)
- Average follow-up 2.4 years
- Standardized anteroposterior and frog-leg lateral radiographs were obtained at baseline and at follow-up.
- Hip measurements
  ▷ Alpha angle
  ▷ Anterosuperior head–neck junction classified by a 3-point visual system

▷ Normal: Slight symmetric concavities of the anterior head–neck junction compared to posterior head–neck junction

▷ Flattened: Moderate decrease in the anterior head–neck offset compared to posterior head–neck junction

▷ Presence of a prominence: A convexity, as opposed to a concavity, in the anterior head–neck junction

▷ Growth plate extension into the neck

▷ Neck-shaft angle

▶ Amount of internal hip rotation measured clinically

▶ Differences between baseline and follow-up radiographic values calculated

▶ Follow-up radiographs reviewed in a randomized order by observers blinded to baseline data

Results

▶ Overall, there was a significant increase in the prevalence of a cam deformity during follow-up.

▷ Of 64 hips that had normal appearance of the anterosuperior head–neck junction at baseline, 35 developed either a flattening or prominence at follow-up.

▶ In boys ages 12 and 13 years at baseline, the prevalence of a flattened head–neck junction increased significantly during follow-up (13.6% to 50.0%; $P = 0.002$).

▶ In all hips with an open growth plate at baseline, the prevalence of a prominence increased from 2.1% to 17.7% ($P = 0.002$).

▶ After proximal femoral growth plate closure, there was no significant increase in the prevalence or increase in severity of a cam deformity.

▶ Alpha angle increased significantly from 59.4 degrees at baseline to 61.3 degrees at follow-up ($P = 0.018$)

▶ The amount of growth plate extension was significantly associated with the alpha angle and hip classification ($P = 0.001$).

▶ A small neck-shaft angle and limited internal rotation were associated with cam deformities and could also significantly predict the formation of cam deformities (α angle > 60 degrees) at follow-up.

Conclusions

▶ In youth soccer players, cam deformities gradually develop during skeletal maturation and probably only during skeletal growth.

▶ Formation of a cam deformity is probably the result of frequent high-impact sports activities that biomechanically trigger extra bone formation at the anterolateral head–neck junction.

▶ Cam deformity formation might be prevented by adjusting athletic activities during a small period of skeletal growth, which will have a major effect on the prevalence of hip osteoarthritis.

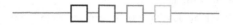

FEATURED ARTICLE

Authors: Philippon MJ, Wolff AB, Briggs KK, Zehms CT, Kuppersmith DA.

Title: Acetabular rim reduction for the treatment of femoroacetabular impingement correlates with preoperative and post-operative center-edge angle.

Journal Information: *Arthroscopy.* 2010;26:757–761.

Study Design: Cohort Study

▶ Study purpose: To quantify the change in degrees in the center-edge (CE) angle for each millimeter of acetabular rim resected in hips undergoing arthroscopic acetabular rim trimming.

Methods

▶ Preoperative and post-operative CE angle and mm of rim reduction were prospectively collected in 58 hips that underwent arthroscopic rim reduction.
▶ Mean patient age 32 years (18 to 61 years), 35 women, 23 men
▶ Inclusion criterion: Hip arthroscopy for FAI in patients without dysplastic hips
▶ 2 orthopedic surgeons made independent measurements of the CE angle on preoperative and post-operative anteroposterior pelvis radiographs.
▶ To determine the amount of rim reduction intraoperatively, the lunate surface was measured with an arthroscopic ruler at the 12 o'clock position before and after rim trimming.

Results

▶ The mean rim reduction performed was 3.2 mm (1 to 9 mm).
▶ Mean change in CE angle was 3.9 degrees (0 to 17 degrees).

- Interobserver intraclass correlation coefficient for radiographic measurement of the CE angle was 0.92 (95% confidence interval, 0.87 to 0.95), indicating excellent interobserver reliability.
- Using a regression model, the change in the CE angle could be determined by the following formula:
  - Change in CE angle = 1.8 + (0.64 × rim reduction in millimeters)

Conclusions

- The amount of change in CE angle can be estimated by the amount of bony resection performed at the 12 o'clock position on the lunate surface in the arthroscopic treatment of FAI.
- 1 mm of bony resection equals 2.4 degrees of change in the CE angle, and 5 mm of bony resection equals 5 degrees of change in the CE angle.
- Change in CE angle = 1.8 + (0.64 × rim reduction in millimeters)

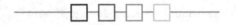

FEATURED ARTICLE

Authors: Bedi A, Dolan M, Hetsroni I, Magennis E, Lipman J, Buly R, Kelly BT.

Title: Surgical treatment of femoroacetabular impingement improves hip kinematics: a computer-assisted model.

Journal Information: *Am J Sports Med.* 2011;39 Suppl:43S–49S.

Study Design: Cohort Study

- Study purpose: To assess differences in hip ROM before and after the arthroscopic surgical treatment of symptomatic FAI using computer-assisted 3-dimensional (3D) analysis.

Methods

- 10 patients with symptomatic, focal cam, and/or pincer impingement lesions
- High-resolution computed tomography (CT) scans and computer-assisted 3D modeling of the hip performed before and after corrective arthroscopic surgery

- ▶ Cam location, alpha angle, neck-shaft angle, femoral version, and acetabular version at 12 o'clock through 3 o'clock positions were measured.
- ▶ Model dynamized to define the preop and post-op ROM and location of impingement with hip flexion and internal rotation at 90 degrees of hip flexion

Results

- ▶ The cam lesion was located between 12 o'clock and 5 o'clock in all cases.
- ▶ Mean preop alpha angle 59.8 degrees (36 to 76 degrees)
- ▶ Mean femoral version 12.5 degrees (−15 to 32 degrees)
- ▶ Mean preoperative hip flexion 107.4 degrees ± 11.6 degrees
- ▶ Mean internal rotation at 90 degrees of hip flexion 19.1 degrees ± 13.0 degrees
- ▶ Impingement location was unique in each case and not predictable based on simple radiographic measures such as the alpha angle
- ▶ Significant improvement with corrective femoral and rim
  - ▷ Mean hip flexion improvement 3.8 degrees ($P = 0.002$)
  - ▷ Mean internal rotation improvement 9.3 degrees ($P = 0.0002$)
  - ▷ Mean post-operative alpha angle 36.4 degrees (22 to 46 degrees)

Conclusions

- ▶ Focal cam and/or rim osteoplasty reliably improves hip kinematics and ROM, especially the limitation of internal rotation in a flexed position.
- ▶ Computer tomography–based computer modeling can localize regions of anticipated mechanical impingement in symptomatic FAI patients.
- ▶ A complete osteoplasty in the area of anticipated mechanical impingement predictably improves ROM and may help eliminate the recurrent mechanical impact and secondary chondral injury associated with FAI.

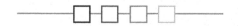

REVIEW ARTICLES

Lavigne M, Parvizi J, Beck M, Siebenrock KA, Ganz R, Leunig M. Anterior femoroacetabular impingement. Part 1. Techniques of joint preserving surgery. *Clin Orthop.* 2004;418:61–66.

Nepple JJ, Prather H, Trousdale RT, et al. Clinical diagnosis of femoroacetabular impingement. *J Am Acad Orthop Surg.* 2013;21:S16–S19.

Sankar WN, Nevitt M, Parvizi J, Felson DT, Agricola R, Leunig M. Femoroacetabular impingement: defining the condition and its role in the pathophysiology of osteoarthritis. *J Am Acad Orthop Surg.* 2013;21:S7–S15.

An excellent review of FAI surgical techniques.

Byrd JWT. Femoroacetabular impingement in athletes: current concepts. *Am J Sports Med.* 2014;42:737–751.

Miscellaneous Hip Topics

FEATURED ARTICLE

Authors: Ilizaliturri VM Jr, Chaidez C, Villegas P, Briseño A, Camacho-Galindo J.

Title: Prospective randomized study of 2 different techniques for endoscopic iliopsoas tendon release in the treatment of internal snapping hip syndrome.

Journal Information: *Arthroscopy.* 2009;25:159–163.

Study Design: Prospective Randomized Study

▸ 19 patients with internal snapping hip syndrome
▸ Randomized to:
  ▷ Endoscopic iliopsoas tendon release at the lesser trochanter (10 patients)
    » Average age 29.5 years, 5 men, 5 women
  ▷ Endoscopic transcapsular psoas release (9 patients)
    » Average age 32.6 years, 8 women, 1 man
▸ Hip arthroscopy was performed in both groups, and associated injuries were identified and treated.
▸ Both treatment groups received the same post-op physical therapy along with 400 mg of celecoxib daily for 21 days after surgery.
▸ Average follow-up 20 months, all with a minimum 12-month follow-up

Miller MD, Mauffrey C, Hak DJ.
*Rapid Reference Review in Sports Medicine:
Pivotal Papers Revealed (pp 163-177).*
© 2016 Taylor & Francis Group.

▶ Assessment
  ▷ Western Ontario and McMaster Universities Arthritis Index (WOMAC)
    scores

Results

▶ The snapping phenomenon was successfully treated in every patient in both
  groups.
▶ WOMAC scores
  ▷ Iliopsoas tendon release at the lesser trochanter
    » 70.1 preop
    » 83.7 at follow-up ($P = 0.001$)
  ▷ Transcapsular psoas release from the peripheral compartment
    » 67 preop
    » 83.6 at follow-up ($P = 0.001$)
▶ No statistical difference between groups in preop WOMAC scores ($P = 0.55$)
▶ Improvements in WOMAC scores were statistically significant in both
  groups ($P = 0.001$).
▶ No difference was found in post-op WOMAC results between groups
  ($P = 0.039$).
▶ No complications

Conclusion

▶ Iliopsoas tendon release at the level of the lesser trochanter or at the level
  of the hip joint using a transcapsular technique is equally effective and
  reproducible.

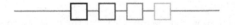

FEATURED ARTICLE

Authors: Gautier E, Ganz K, Krügel N, Gill T, Ganz R.

Title: Anatomy of the medial femoral circumflex artery and its surgical implications.

Journal Information: *J Bone Joint Surg Br.* 2000;82:679–683.

Study Design: Cadaveric Study

▶ Purpose: To investigate the course of the medial femoral circumflex and its topographical relationship to the tendons of the external rotators and the hip capsule, and to investigate the effect of surgical hip dislocation on the vessel

▶ Dissected 24 hips after neoprene-latex injection into the femoral or internal iliac artery

▶ 5 consistent branches of the medial femoral circumflex artery

▷ Superficial branch courses between pectineus and adductor longus

▷ Ascending branch courses to adductor brevis, adductor magnus, and obturator externus

▷ Acetabular branch gives off the foveolar artery (medial epiphyseal artery)

▷ Descending branch courses between quadratus femoris and adductor magnus, supplying the ischiocrural muscles

▷ Deep branch courses to the femoral head

Results

▶ The course of the deep branch of the medial femoral circumflex artery was constant in its extracapsular segment.

▶ A trochanteric branch was present in all cases at the proximal border of quadratus femoris, spreading onto the lateral aspect of the greater trochanter.

▶ The trochanteric branch marks the level of the tendon of obturator externus, which is crossed posteriorly by the deep branch of the medial femoral circumflex artery.

▶ As the deep branch travels superiorly, it crosses anterior to the conjoint tendon of the inferior gemellus, obturator internus, and superior gemellus.

▶ The deep branch then perforates the joint capsule at the level of the superior gemellus.

▶ The intracapsular segment of the deep branch runs along the posterosuperior aspect of the femoral neck, dividing into 2 to 4 subsynovial retinacular vessels.

▶ The obturator externus protects the deep branch of the medial femoral circumflex artery from disruption or stretching during hip dislocation after serial release of all other soft tissue attachments of the proximal femur, including a complete circumferential capsulotomy.

▶ Despite prior descriptions, they found no anastomotic branch surrounding the cranial aspect of the femoral neck that communicated with the ascending branch of the lateral femoral circumflex artery.

▶ They found a significant constant anastomosis between the medial femoral circumflex artery and a branch of the inferior gluteal artery along the piriformis, which may be capable of compensating after injury to the deep branch of the medial femoral circumflex artery.

Conclusions

▶ The deep branch of the medial femoral circumflex artery is the primary blood supply of the femoral head.

▶ The short external rotators are often divided in posterior approaches to the hip and pelvis, which can damage the deep branch and interfere with femoral head perfusion.

▶ The deep branch of the medial femoral circumflex artery can be damaged when retractors leave the posteromedial area proximal to the lesser trochanter unprotected.

▶ Knowledge of the medial femoral circumflex artery extracapsular anatomy is necessary to avoid iatrogenic femoral head avascular necrosis in reconstructive surgery of the hip and open reduction of acetabular fractures through the posterior Kocher-Langenbeck approach.

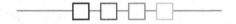

FEATURED ARTICLE

Authors: Draovitch P, Edelstein J, Kelly BT.

Title: The layer concept: utilization in determining the pain generators, pathology and how structure determines treatment.

Journal Information: *Curr Rev Musculoskelet Med.* 2012;5:1–8.

▶ This paper outlines the layer concept, developed by Dr. Bryan Kelly, which is a systematic means of determining which structures about nonarthritic hips are the source of the pathology and which are the pain generators.

▶ Deciphering the etiology of the pathology vs the pain generator is essential in selecting the proper treatment.

▶ 4 layers described

  ▷ Layer I: Osteochondral layer

    » Consists of the femur, pelvis, and acetabulum.

    » This layer's purpose is to offer joint congruence and structurally guide normal kinematics.

    » Developmental-related pathologies include dysplasia, femoral version, acetabular version, femoral inclination, and acetabular profunda/protrusion.

- » Dynamic-related pathologies include cam/pincer impingement, trochanteric impingement, subspine impingement, and delamination.
- ▷ Layer II: Inert tissue layer
  - » Consists of the labrum, capsule, ligamentous complex, and ligamentum teres
  - » This layer's purpose is to provide static stability to the joint.
  - » Pathologies include labral tears, ligamentum teres tear, capsular instability, ligament tears, and adhesive capsulitis.
- ▷ Layer III: Contractile layer
  - » Consists of all contractile tissues that support, control, and move the hip joint, including trunk stabilizers and pelvic floor musculature
  - » This layer's purpose is to provide dynamic stability to the hip, pelvis, and trunk.
  - » Pathologies include psoas impingement, rectus femoris impingement, gluteus medius and minimus tears, hip flexor strain, and various enthesiopathies and tendinopathies.
- ▷ Layer IV: Neuromechanical layer
  - » Consists of anatomic structures, physiologic events, and kinematic factors that drive proprioception and pain within the hip, including neurovascular structures, mechanoreceptors, nociceptors, and thorocolumbar and lower extremity mechanics
  - » Pathologies include nerve entrapment, referred spinal pathology, neuromuscular dysfunction, and pain syndromes.
- ▸ This paper also describes special tests that may be used for each layer.
- ▸ Clinical treatment of hip pain is guided by the examination and begins from layer IV and progresses in toward layer I.

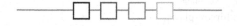

FEATURED ARTICLE

Authors: Clohisy JC, Nepple JJ, Larson CM, Zaltz I, Millis M.

Title: Persistent structural disease is the most common cause of repeat hip preservation surgery.

Journal Information: *Clin Orthop Relat Res.* 2013;471:3788–3794.

Study Design: Cohort Study

▶ Study purposes

  ▷ To characterize patients undergoing hip preservation surgery after prior procedures

  ▷ To compare demographics, hip pain, and function in patients with prior procedures with those undergoing primary surgery

  ▷ To determine the types of previous procedures and the reasons for secondary surgery

  ▷ To report the procedure profile of the secondary surgeries

Methods

▶ A prospective, multicenter hip preservation database (Academic Network of Conservation Hip Outcome Research—ANCHOR) of 2263 patients (2386 surgery cases) was queried from January 1, 2007 to September 5, 2012.

▶ Three hundred fifty-three patients (359 hips) identified who had prior surgery

▶ All patients had persistent or recurrent symptoms after their initial surgery.

▶ Patient demographics, type of previous surgery, diagnostic categories, clinical scores, and type of secondary procedure were recorded.

▶ Baseline clinical scores

  ▷ Modified Harris Hip Score

  ▷ WOMAC

  ▷ SF-12

▶ Patients were subclassified into 5 categories based on diagnoses assigned at the time of secondary surgery

  ▷ Femoroacetabular impingement (FAI)/labral tears

  ▷ Adult hip dysplasia

  ▷ Pediatric hip dysplasia

  ▷ Slipped capital femoral epiphysis

  ▷ Legg-Calve-Perthes disease/residual Perthes-like deformities

Results

▶ Average patient age at secondary surgery 23 years (10 to 54 years), 249 women, 104 men

▶ Mean number of prior surgeries 1.1, 12% of hips had > 1 prior surgery

▶ Hip pain and function were similar between patients undergoing primary and secondary surgery.

▶ Patients undergoing secondary surgery were more frequently female and had a younger average age than those having no prior hip surgery.

▶ Prior surgical approaches were open in 52% and hip arthroscopy in 48%.

▶ In the FAI subgroup, hip arthroscopy was the most common previous surgical approach (86%).

▶ In the adult acetabular dysplasia subgroup, hip arthroscopy was the most common previous surgical approach (64%).

▶ Secondary hip preservation procedures were performed using:

▷ Open approach (72%)

▷ Arthroscopic approach (21%)

▷ Combined arthroscopic and open approach (7%)

▶ Inadequately corrected structural disease was the most common reason for secondary surgery.

▶ Femoral osteochondroplasty, labral procedures, and acetabular reorientation were common secondary procedures.

▶ Secondary procedures performed (% of 359 hips that procedure was performed)

▷ Femoral head–neck osteochondroplasty (74%)

▷ Labral procedure (refixation/debridement) (45%)

▷ Periacetabular osteotomy (25%)

▷ Acetabular articular cartilage procedure (21%)

▷ Acetabular rim trimming (20%)

▷ Femoral head articular cartilage procedure (8%)

▷ Femoral osteotomy (6%)

Conclusions

▶ Inadequately corrected structural disease (FAI or acetabular dysplasia) was commonly associated with the need for secondary hip preservation surgery.

▶ Although the authors did not have data to identify other technical failures, the available data suggest primary treatments should encompass comprehensive deformity correction when indicated.

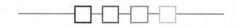

FEATURED ARTICLE

Authors: de Sa D, Alradwan H, Cargnelli S, Thawer Z, Simunovic N, Cadet E, Bonin N, Larson C, Ayeni OR.

Title: Extra-articular hip impingement: a systematic review examining operative treatment of psoas, subspine, ischiofemoral, and greater trochanteric/pelvic impingement.

Journal Information: *Arthroscopy.* 2014;30:1026–1041.

Study Design: Systematic Review

▸ Extra-articular hip impingement can result from:
  ▷ Psoas impingement
  ▷ Subspine impingement
  ▷ Ischiofemoral impingement
  ▷ Greater trochanteric/pelvic impingement
▸ Symptoms may be due to bony abutment or soft tissue irritation, and it is often challenging to differentiate among symptoms preoperatively.
▸ This systematic review was conducted to examine each condition and elucidate the surgical indications, treatment options, and clinical outcomes.

Methods

▸ MEDLINE, EMBASE, and PUBMED databases searched for English-language clinical studies addressing the surgical treatment of psoas impingement, subspine impingement, ischiofemoral impingement, and greater trochanteric/pelvic impingement.
▸ For each condition, 2 independent assessors reviewed eligible studies.
▸ 9521 studies were initially retrieved and ultimately 14 studies examining 333 hips were included.

Results

▸ Psoas impingement
  ▷ Arthroscopic surgery resulted in 88% of patients achieving good to excellent results.
  ▷ Significant improvement in the Harris Hip Score ($P = 0.008$)
  ▷ Significant improvement in Hip Outcome Score—Activities of Daily Living ($P = 0.02$)
  ▷ Significant improvement in Hip Outcome Score—Sport ($P = 0.04$)

- Subspine impingement
  - ▷ Arthroscopic decompression, with no major complications, resulted in a mean 18.5-degree improvement in flexion.
  - ▷ Improvement in pain (mean preop visual analog scale 5.9 points, post-op 1.2 points)
  - ▷ Improvement in modified Harris Hip Score (mean preop score 64.97 points, post-op 91.3 points)
- Ischiofemoral impingement and greater trochanteric/pelvic impingement
  - ▷ Open procedures anecdotally improved patient symptoms, but no formal objective outcomes data were reported.

Conclusions

- There is some evidence to support that arthroscopic treatment of psoas impingement and subspine impingement results in improved patient outcomes.
- There is some evidence to support that open surgical treatment of ischiofemoral impingement and greater trochanteric/pelvic impingement results in improved patient outcomes.

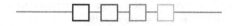

FEATURED ARTICLE

Authors: Harris JD, McCormick FM, Abrams GD, Gupta AK, Ellis TJ, Bach BR Jr, Bush-Joseph CA, Nho SJ.

Title: Complications and reoperations during and after hip arthroscopy: a systematic review of 92 studies and more than 6000 patients.

Journal Information: *Arthroscopy*. 2013;29:589–595.

Study Design: Systematic Review

- Purpose: To determine the prevalence of complications and reoperations during and after hip arthroscopy

Methods

- A systematic review of multiple MEDLINE, SciVerse Scopus, SportDiscus, and Cochrane Central Register of Controlled Trials databases was performed.

▶ All clinical outcome studies that reported the presence or absence of complications and/or reoperations were eligible for inclusion.

▶ 961 potentially relevant studies identified and screened

▶ 92 studies (6134 patients) were included in final analysis

▶ Most were level IV evidence studies (88%) with short-term follow-up (mean follow-up 2.0 years).

▶ Duplicate patient populations within separate distinct publications were analyzed and reported only once.

▶ Preferred Reporting Items for Systematic Reviews and Meta-Analyses (PRISMA) guidelines and checklist used

▶ Complication and reoperation rates were extracted from each study.

Results

▶ Labral tears and FAI were the 2 most common diagnoses treated.

▶ Labral treatment and acetabuloplasty/femoral osteochondroplasty were the 2 most common surgical techniques reported.

▶ 0.58% (37) overall rate of major complications

   ▷ Damage to perineal skin, hip dislocation, intra-abdominal and intrathoracic fluid extravasation, hypothermia, infection, thromboembolism, avascular necrosis, heterotopic ossification, femoral neck fracture, and death all occurred at a rate of < 1%.

▶ 7.5% (479) overall rate of minor complications

   ▷ Iatrogenic chondrolabral injury and temporary neuropraxia were the 2 most common minor complications.

▶ 6.3% overall reoperation rate, occurring at a mean of 16 months

▶ Total hip arthroplasty (THA) was the most common reoperation.

▶ 2.9% conversion rate to THA

Conclusions

▶ The most common reason for reoperation was conversion to THA (conversion rate 2.9%).

▶ As surgical indications evolve, patient selection should limit the number of cases that would have been converted to THA.

▶ Minor complications and reoperation rate are directly related to the hip arthroscopy learning curve.

▶ The number of future minor complications is expected to decrease with increased surgeon experience and instrumentation improvements.

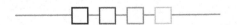

FEATURED ARTICLE

Authors: Philippon MJ, Briggs KK, Carlisle JC, Patterson DC.

Title: Joint space predicts THA after hip arthroscopy in patients 50 years and older.

Journal Information: *Clin Orthop Relat Res.* 2013;471:2492–2496.

Study Design: Cohort Study

▶ The degree of radiographic osteoarthritis predicts subsequent THA in patients considering joint-preserving hip arthroscopy.

▶ Purpose: To identify the best radiographic measure that predicts THA after hip arthroscopy.

Methods

▶ Retrospectively reviewed 203 patients ≥50 years of age treated with hip arthroscopy between March 2007 and October 2010

▶ Data were collected prospectively and retrospectively analyzed.

▶ Inclusion criteria: complete quality radiographs, radiographic diagnosis of FAI, prospectively collected radiographic measurements, preoperative modified Harris Hip Score, and minimum 3 years post–hip arthroscopy

▶ 96 patients met the study inclusion criteria.

   ▷ 31 patients underwent THA during the follow-up time.

   ▷ 65 patients did not undergo THA.

   » Median follow-up of patients not undergoing THA 54 months

▶ Average age at time of hip arthroscopy 57 years (50 to 78 years), 49 men, 47 women

▶ Examined 3 radiographic features prior to arthroscopy

   ▷ Tönnis grade

   ▷ Kellgren-Lawrence grade

   ▷ Joint-space narrowing measured at 3 locations

   » Lateral edge of the sourcil

   » Middle of the sourcil

   » In line with the fovea

Results

▶ Characteristics of patients who underwent THA and who did not were similar.

▶ The only factor that was different between the 2 groups was more patients in the THA group than the non-THA group ($P = 0.001$) underwent acetabular microfractures.

▶ Patients with ≤2 mm of joint space were 12 times (95% confidence interval, 5 to 34) more likely to undergo THA than patients with >2 mm of joint space.

▶ Joint space (≤2 mm) predicted THA in 81% of the patients.

▶ There was an association between subsequent THA and the Kellgren-Lawrence grade ($P = 0.003$) and Tönnis grade ($P = 0.002$).

▶ Patients with Tönnis grade of 2 or 3 were 4.8 times (95% confidence interval, 1.8 to 12.6) more likely to require THA.

▶ Patients with Kellgren-Lawrence grade 3 or 4 were 4.8 times (95% confidence interval, 2.0 to 11.3) more likely to require THA.

▶ Kellgren-Lawrence grade 3 or 4 predicted THA in 73% of the patients.

▶ Tönnis grade 2 or 3 predicted THA in 65% of patients and had the lowest accuracy.

▶ On binary logistic regression, the only predictor ($r^2 = 0.45$) of THA was joint space of 2 mm or less.

Conclusions

▶ Measuring joint space by determining if any measurement is 2 mm or less predicts patients progressing to THA after hip arthroscopy approximately 80% of the time.

▶ At the time that hip arthroscopy is considered, joint-space measurements were the most accurate predictor of subsequent need for THA and should be used in patient education to define the risk of early failure from hip arthroscopy.

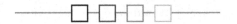

FEATURED ARTICLE

Authors: Walters BL, Cooper JH, Rodriguez JA.

Title: New findings in hip capsular anatomy: dimensions of capsular thickness and pericapsular contributions.

Journal Information: *Arthroscopy.* 2014;30:1235–1245.

Study Design: Cadaveric Study

▶ Study purpose: To provide a detailed description of the anatomy of the hip capsule and pericapsular structures.

Methods

▶ Dissected 11 nonpaired, fresh-frozen cadaveric hips

▶ Documentation of capsular thickness, origins, insertions, and attachments to pericapsular structures, including the abductors, rectus femoris, piriformis, short external rotators, and iliocapsularis muscles, performed by 2 independent observers

▶ Tendinous insertions of the surrounding pericapsular muscles were measured according to size and distance from reproducible osseous landmarks.

Results

▶ The hip capsule originates at a mean 5.1 mm proximal and medial to the bony rim of the acetabulum, creating a small intracapsular recess (recess smallest anterosuperiorly and largest posteriorly).

▶ Near the acetabular origin the capsule is thickest superiorly and posterosuperiorly (3.7 to 4.0 mm).

▶ The capsule is thinnest anteriorly and anteroinferiorly (1.3 mm).

▶ The iliocapsularis, indirect head of the rectus, conjoint, obturator externus, and gluteus minimus tendons all show consistent capsular contributions.

▶ In contrast, the piriformis does not have a capsular attachment.

▶ The inter-relation of these structures is complex, yet their relations to the anterior hip capsule and contributions to its thickness are predictable.

Conclusions

▶ The static and dynamic pericapsular hip structures are intimately associated and contribute to reproducible patterns of anterior capsular thickness.

▶ The dynamic pericapsular structures include the iliocapsularis, gluteus minimus, and reflected head of the rectus femoris.

▶ The static stabilizers of the hip include the iliofemoral, ischiofemoral, and pubofemoral ligaments.

▶ At the acetabulum, the thickest region of the capsule is posterosuperior and superolateral.

▶ At the femoral insertion, the thickest region is anterior.

▶ Understanding the intricate relation between the hip capsule and pericapsular structures is useful for surgeons who perform the precise and specific capsular releases required during hip arthroscopy.

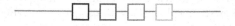

FEATURED ARTICLE

Authors: Philippon MJ, Michalski MP, Campbell KJ, Goldsmith MT, Devitt BM, Wijdicks CA, LaPrade RF.

Title: An anatomical study of the acetabulum with clinical applications to hip arthroscopy.

Journal Information: *J Bone Joint Surg Am.* 2014;96:1673–1682.

Study Design: Cadaveric Study

▶ Study purpose: To qualitatively and quantitatively describe arthroscopically relevant anatomy of the acetabulum with an aim to present a surgical landmark that is located in close proximity to the usual location of labral pathology as an alternative to the midpoint of the transverse acetabular ligament as a reference point.

Methods

▶ 14 fresh-frozen cadaveric hemipelves were dissected to evaluate osseous landmarks and relevant surrounding soft tissue structures of the acetabulum.

▶ Used a coordinate-measuring device to determine the location, orientation, and relationship of key arthroscopic landmarks and the footprint areas of the insertions of the rectus femoris, capsule, and labrum.

Results

▶ The superior margin of the anterior labral sulcus (psoas-u) was the most consistent anatomic landmark based on analysis of variability of reference points around the acetabulum in relation to the anterior inferior iliac spine (AIIS).

▶ The AIIS consists of superior and inferior facets, demarcated by the origins of the rectus femoris direct head and iliocapsularis.

▶ The inferolateral aspect of the rectus femoris direct head footprint was 19.2 mm from the acetabular rim (95% confidence interval, 18.0 to 20.4 mm).

▶ The inferolateral aspect of the iliocapsularis footprint was 12.5 mm from the acetabular rim (95% confidence interval, 10.1 to 15.0 mm).

Conclusions

▶ The superior margin of the anterior labral sulcus (psoas-u) was a reliable landmark for reference of the clock face on the acetabulum.

▶ The authors propose that this point, denoting 3 o'clock, be adopted as the new standard clock-face reference for intra-articular hip structures because of its universal presence and reliable arthroscopic visualization.

▶ This marker is also beneficial because of its proximity to the typical location of labral pathology.

▶ The establishment of a new standard reference point within the acetabulum will serve to increase the consistency of labral pathology location identification and improve arthroscopic orientation and navigation.

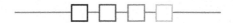

REVIEW ARTICLE

Shu B, Safran MR. Hip instability: anatomic and clinical considerations of traumatic and atraumatic instability. *Clin Sports Med*. 2011;30:349–367.

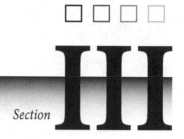

Shoulder

Shoulder Anatomy, Biomechanics, and Clinical Rating Systems

Chapter **16**

FEATURED ARTICLE
Authors: Constant CR, Murley AHG.
Title: A clinical method of functional assessment of the shoulder.
Journal Information: *Clin Orthop Rel Res*. 1987;214:160–164.

▶ This paper describes the Constant scoring system.

▶ The authors emphasize that the method is applicable irrespective of the details of the diagnostic or radiologic abnormalities caused by disease or injury.

▶ It is reproducible by different observers.

▶ It is sufficiently sensitive to reveal even small changes in function.

▶ The system is based on a 100-point scale.

  ▷ Subjective parameters

    » Pain assessment—15 possible points

    » Activities of daily living—20 possible points

  ▷ Objective parameters

    » Range of motion—40 possible points

    » Power using a Cybex II Dynamometer—25 possible points

▶ Low index of observer error

  ▷ 3 observers assessed 100 shoulders.

  ▷ Average 3% observer error (0% to 8%)

Miller MD, Mauffrey C, Hak DJ.
*Rapid Reference Review in Sports Medicine:
Pivotal Papers Revealed (pp 181-194).*
© 2016 Taylor & Francis Group.

- The authors concluded that the quantification of shoulder disability is not feasible.
- Their scoring system allows:
  - Establishment of a normal level of shoulder function appropriate to different age groups
  - Establishment of what constitutes a disability
  - Assessment of the differential rates of progress following treatment of an injury or disease

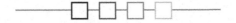

FEATURED ARTICLE

Authors: Harryman DT 2nd, Sidles JA, Harris SL, Matsen FA 3rd.

Title: The role of the rotator interval capsule in passive motion and stability of the shoulder.

Journal Information: *J Bone Joint Surg Am.* 1992;74:53–66.

Study Design: Cadaveric Study

- Purpose: To characterize the role of the capsule in the interval between the supraspinatus and subscapularis tendons with respect to glenohumeral motion, translation, and stability.
- Studied 8 cadaveric shoulders
- 6-degrees-of-freedom position sensor and 6-degrees-of-freedom force and torque transducer used to determine the glenohumeral rotations and translations that resulted from applied loads
- Range of motion of each specimen was measured with:
  - Capsule in the rotator interval in a normal state
  - After the capsule had been sectioned
  - After the capsule had been imbricated
- Passive stability of the glenohumeral joint was evaluated with the use of anterior, posterior, and inferior stress tests.

Results

- Alteration of this capsular interval affected flexion, extension, external rotation, and adduction of the humerus with respect to the scapula.

- ▶ Modification of this portion of the capsule also affected obligate anterior translation of the humeral head on the glenoid during flexion
    - ▷ 12.3 mm ± 4.0 mm with intact capsule
    - ▷ 8.9 mm ± 4.3 mm with sectioned capsule
    - ▷ 18.0 mm ± 3.6 mm with imbricated capsule
- ▶ Limitation of motion and obligate translation were increased by imbrication and decreased by sectioning of the rotator interval capsule.
- ▶ Instability and occasional frank dislocation of the glenohumeral joint occurred inferiorly and posteriorly after section of the rotator interval capsule.
- ▶ Imbrication of this part of the capsule increased the resistance to inferior and posterior translation.

Conclusions and Clinical Relevance

- ▶ This study suggests that the capsule in the rotator interval plays an important role in glenohumeral motion and stability.
- ▶ Release of this part of the capsule may improve the range of motion of shoulders that have limited flexion and external rotation.
- ▶ Imbrication of the rotator interval capsule may help to control posterior and inferior instability.

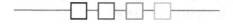

FEATURED ARTICLE

Authors: Brooks CH, Revel WJ, Heatley FW.

Title: A quantitative histologic study of the vascularity of the rotator cuff tendon.

Journal Information: *J Bone Joint Surg Br.* 1992;74:151–153.

Study Design: Cadaveric Study

- ▶ The cause of rotator cuff rupture has been debated, and various etiologic factors (hypovascularity, degeneration, trauma, and impingement) have been proposed.
- ▶ In 1934 Codman described the distal 10 mm of the supraspinatus tendon as a "critical zone" since it is the most common site for cuff tears.

- Because supraspinatus tears occur most frequently in Codman's "critical zone," many surgeons considered hypovascularity to be a major etiologic factor.
- Prior cadaveric perfusion studies have demonstrated that this area is "hypovascular."
- Other histologic studies have indicated that the entire tendon is well vascularized, but that vessels can become occluded with abduction.
- 8 cadavers ages 62 to 78 were perfused with barium and fixed in formalin to study the rotator cuff vasculature.
- Quantitative histologic analysis was performed at 5-mm intervals from the humeral insertions to the muscle bellies.
  - ▷ Vessel number
  - ▷ Vessel size
  - ▷ Percentage of tendon occupied by vessels

Results

- The distal 15 mm of both the supraspinatus and infraspinatus tendons was hypovascular.
- No significant difference between the vascularity of supraspinatus and the infraspinatus
- Number of vessels and mean vessel diameter decreased toward the humeral insertion of the supraspinatus tendon.
- The decrease in the percentage of the tendon occupied by vessels was most marked between 10 and 20 mm from its humeral insertion ($P < 0.01$).

Conclusions

- Investigators found no difference in the vascular pattern between infraspinatus and supraspinatus tendons, implying that other factors are more important in the tendon rupture pathogenesis.
- If vascularity was the major etiologic factor, then one would expect the incidence of supraspinatus and infraspinatus ruptures to be similar.
- Therefore, factors other than vascularity are important in the pathogenesis of supraspinatus rupture.

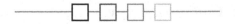

FEATURED ARTICLE

Authors: Turkel SJ, Panio MW, Marshall JL, Girgis FG.

Title: Stabilizing mechanisms preventing anterior dislocation of the glenohumeral joint.

Journal Information: *J Bone Joint Surg Am.* 1981;63:1208–1217.

Study Design: Cadaveric Study

▶ Purpose: To identify what each periarticular structure contributes to the stability of the glenohumeral joint.

▶ 36 embalmed cadaveric specimens dissected to study the stabilizing mechanism of the glenohumeral joint that prevents anterior dislocation
  ▷ Subscapularis
  ▷ Shoulder capsule
  ▷ Superior glenohumeral ligament
  ▷ Middle glenohumeral ligament
  ▷ Inferior glenohumeral ligament

▶ The relative importance of each of these structures in limiting external rotation in various shoulder positions by cutting them serially in different sequences.

▶ Radiographic studies also performed in 10 unembalmed cadaveric shoulders in which radiopaque markers were used to demonstrate the position, tightness, and laxity of the subscapularis muscle and of the middle and inferior glenohumeral ligaments during external rotation of the shoulder at 0, 45, and 90 degrees of abduction.

▶ The subscapularis muscle and the three glenohumeral ligaments were cut in different sequences to determine their relative contributions to stability (limitation of external rotation).

Results

▶ After cutting the subscapularis muscle, external rotation increased:
  ▷ 15 to 20 degrees (average 18 degrees) at 0 degrees of abduction
  ▷ 5 to 17 degrees (average 9 degrees) at 45 degrees of abduction
  ▷ 1 to 11 degrees (average 3 degrees) at 90 degrees of abduction

- After cutting the superior glenohumeral ligament (in addition to the subscapularis), the further increase in external rotation was relatively small.
  - ▷ 2 to 11 degrees (average 5 degrees) at 0 degrees of abduction
  - ▷ 1 to 4 degrees (average 2 degrees) at 45 degrees of abduction
  - ▷ 1 to 6 degrees (average 2 degrees) at 90 degrees of abduction
- After cutting the middle glenohumeral ligament (in addition to the two above), the further increase in external rotation was:
  - ▷ 3 to 10 degrees (average 5 degrees) at 0 degrees of abduction
  - ▷ 4 to 15 degrees (average 8 degrees) at 45 degrees of abduction
  - ▷ 0 to 1 degree (average 1 degree) at 90 degrees of abduction
- After cutting the superior band of the inferior glenohumeral ligament (in addition to the 3 above), external rotation increased by:
  - ▷ 4 and 8 degrees in 2 specimens, subluxation in 2, and dislocation in 1
  - ▷ 1 to 9 degrees (average 4 degrees) increase at 45 degrees of abduction
  - ▷ 0 to 4 degrees (average 2 degrees) increase at 90 degrees of abduction
- After cutting the anterior portion of the axillary pouch of the inferior glenohumeral ligament (in addition to the 4 structures above), external rotation increased by:
  - ▷ 18 and 32 degrees in 2 specimens, subluxation in 2, and dislocation in 1 at 0 degrees of abduction
  - ▷ 10 to 17 degrees (average 13 degrees) in 3 specimens, subluxation in 1, and dislocation in 1 specimen at 45 degrees of abduction
  - ▷ At 90 degrees of abduction, the shoulder that dislocated at 45 degrees of abduction continued to do so, but the other 4 shoulders showed only minimal increases of external rotation.
- After cutting the posterior region of the axillary pouch, external rotation caused frank dislocation in all 5 specimens in all positions of abduction.

Conclusions

- At 0 degrees of abduction, the subscapularis muscle stabilizes the joint to a large extent.
- At 45 degrees of abduction, the subscapularis, middle glenohumeral ligament, and anterosuperior fibers of the inferior glenohumeral ligament provide the stability.
- As the shoulder approaches 90 degrees of abduction, the inferior glenohumeral ligament prevents dislocation during external rotation.

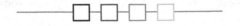

FEATURED ARTICLE

Authors: O'Brien SJ, Neves MC, Arnoczky SP, Rozbruck SR, DiCarlo EF, Warren RF, Schwartz R, Wickiewicz TL.

Title: The anatomy and histology of the inferior glenohumeral ligament complex of the shoulder.

Journal Information: *Am J Sports Med.* 1990;18:449–456.

Study Design: Cadaveric Study

- Purpose: To investigate the gross and histologic anatomy of the inferior glenohumeral ligament in order to describe this structure in detail
- 11 fresh-frozen cadaver shoulders
- Examined arthroscopically
- Joint capsule was then opened and examined; location and shape of the inferior glenohumeral ligament complex attachments to the glenoid and humerus recorded
- Entire joint capsule then completely detached from the glenoid and humerus and processed for histologic examination

Results

- Arthroscopic observations of the joint capsule through the normal range of motion revealed that the inferior glenohumeral ligament is actually a complex of 3 structures (Figure 16-1):
  - Anterior band
  - Posterior band
  - An interposed axillary pouch
- These structures were best demonstrated in some shoulders by placing the humeral head in internal or external rotation with varying degrees of abduction.
- Histologic examination revealed that the anterior and posterior bands of the inferior glenohumeral ligament complex were readily identifiable as distinct structures composed of thickened bands of well-organized collagen bundles.
- The inferior glenohumeral ligament complex was observed to attach to the humeral neck in one of 2 distinct configurations (Figure 16-2):
  - Collarlike attachment, in which the entire inferior glenohumeral ligament complex attaches just inferior to the articular edge of the humeral head

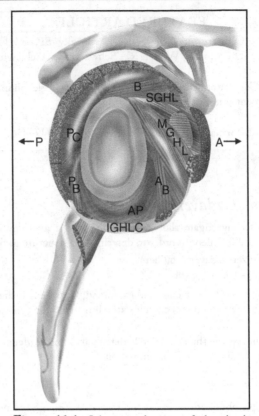

Figure 16-1. Schematic drawing of the shoulder capsule illustrating the location and extent of the IGHLC. (A) anterior; (P) posterior; (B) biceps tendon; (SGHL) superior glenohumeral ligament; (MGHL) middle glenohumeral ligament; (AB) anterior band; (AP) axillary pouch; (PB) posterior band; and (PC) posterior capsule.

▷ V-shaped attachment, with the anterior and posterior bands attaching adjacent to the articular edge of the humeral head and the axillary pouch attaching at the apex of the V distal to the articular edge

Conclusion

▶ The orientation and design of the inferior glenohumeral ligament complex supports the functional concept of this structure as an important anterior and posterior stabilizer of the shoulder joint.

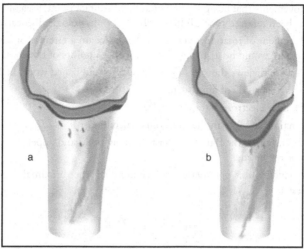

Figure 16-2. Drawings of the proximal humerus illustrating the collar-like (A) and V-shaped (B) attachments of the IGHLC.

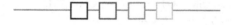

FEATURED ARTICLE

Author: Saha AK.

Title: Mechanics of elevation of the glenohumeral joint.

Journal Information: *Acta Orthop Scan.* 1973;44:668–678.

▸ Author describes the concept of a "zero position" and its applied importance
  ▷ Glenohumeral joint neutral or "zero position" = where there is no further rotation, no active gliding of the joint surfaces and circumduction; where the mechanical axis corresponds to the anatomic axis of the shaft; where gliding, rotation, and "breaststroke" movements become identical
▸ Author outlines the minimum requirements for elevation of the glenohumeral joint without impairment of the dynamic stability
▸ Describes 3 types of shoulder movements:
  ▷ Movement on a fixed contact point, area, or band (hinging) with no change of the mechanical axis

▷ Movements that bring about a change of contact point, area of band—this has been referred to as gliding, rolling, or physiologic dislocation

▷ Movement of rotation, even if it takes place on a circular band contact—pressure would be distributed equally on all points of the contact surface

▶ This article reviews the author's body of prior published work, including:

▷ Cadaveric study of joint surface curvature

▷ Shoulder electromyography studies

▷ Dynamic stability in the horizontal direction

▶ Rehabilitation of the flail shoulder following polio and upper brachial plexus injury is reviewed.

▶ Requirements for prosthetic replacement of the proximal humerus are discussed.

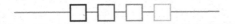

FEATURED ARTICLE

Authors: Harryman DT, Sidles JA, Clark JM, McQuade KJ, Gibb TD, Matsen FA 3rd.

Title: Translation of the humeral head on the glenoid with passive glenohumeral motion.

Journal Information: *J Bone Joint Surg.* 1990;72:1334-1343.

Study Design: Cadaveric Study

▶ Purpose: To examine the direction and magnitude of translations that occur with selected passive motions of isolated shoulder joints and to test the hypothesis that glenohumeral translation is a result of locally tight capsular tissues and not a result of humeral head asphericity.

▶ 7 fresh isolated glenohumeral cadaveric joints with scapula rigidly secured in plaster

▶ Torques and forces applied using a 6-degrees-of-freedom position sensor and 6-axis force transducer

▶ 5 motions studied:

▷ Flexion

▷ Extension

▷ Internal rotation

▷ External rotation
▷ Cross-body movement
▸ Motions studied:
▷ With intact capsule
▷ With capsule vented to air with an 18-gauge needle
▷ After tightening the posterior portion of the capsule (2 cm imbrication of the posterior capsule by mattress suture technique)
▷ After severance of all capsular and tendinous connections between the humerus and scapula (control measurements)

Results

▸ Demonstrated that certain passive motions of the glenohumeral joint are reproducibly accompanied by translation of the humeral head on the glenoid
▸ Reproducible and significant anterior translation occurred with glenohumeral flexion, and posterior translation occurred with glenohumeral extension.
▸ Posterior translation occurred with external rotation.
▸ Anterior translation occurred with cross-body movement.
▸ The anterior translation occurring with flexion was obligate—it could not be prevented by applying an oppositely directed force of 30 to 40 N.
▸ Imbrication of the posterior capsule increased the anterior translation seen with flexion and cross-body movement and caused it to occur earlier in the arc of motion.
▸ Imbrication of the posterior capsule also resulted in significant superior translation with flexion of the glenohumeral joint.

Conclusions and Clinical Significance

▸ Awareness that glenohumeral translation is associated with passive shoulder motion is clinically important in attempts to maintain or restore normal shoulder kinematics.
▸ Translations occurring with passive motions represent a departure from pure ball-and-socket mechanics.
▸ The obligate translations identified in this study are likely to occur during physical examination or physical therapy, when the joint is passively moved to the limits of its motion, resulting in tightening of the capsule.
▸ Glenohumeral translation may also be associated with motion in sports, such as the transition from between the late cocking and early acceleration phases of baseball throwing.
▸ Obligate glenohumeral translations are not the result of ligamentous insufficiency or laxity; instead, they occur when the capsule is asymmetrically tight.

▸ This finding is consistent with the clinical observation that posterior translation is associated with tightness of the anterior capsule, as in osteoarthrosis or
with excessively tight anterior repairs for glenohumeral instability.

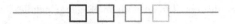

FEATURED ARTICLE

Authors: Warner JJ, Micheli LJ, Arslanian LE, Kennedy J,
Kennedy R.

Title: Scapulothoracic motion in normal shoulders and shoulders
with glenohumeral instability and impingement syndrome.

Journal Information: *Clin Orthop.* 1992;285:199–215.

Study Design: Cohort Study

▸ Normal ratio of glenohumeral to scapulothoracic motion is 2:1.
▸ Qualitative visual inspection and manual muscle testing may overlook subtle
axioscapular muscle weakness.
▸ Used Moiré topographic analysis to assess axioscapular muscle function
  ▷ 22 asymptomatic individuals
  ▷ 22 patients with shoulder instability
  ▷ 7 patients with impingement syndrome
▸ Static assessment
  ▷ Image taken with arms forward and flexed 90 degrees holding a 4.5-kg
    weight in each hand for 5 seconds
▸ Dynamic assessment
  ▷ Lifted 4.5-kg weight in each hand from 0 to 120 degrees in the forward
    plane for 10 repetitions and image taken during the final descent phase
    at approximately 60 to 30 degrees (serratus anterior and trapezius must
    function eccentrically to stabilize the scapula against the chest wall dur-
    ing descent)

Results

- ▶ Rate of scapulothoracic asymmetry or increased topography with static evaluation
  - ▷ 14% of asymptomatic individuals
  - ▷ 32% of patients with shoulder instability
  - ▷ 57% of patients with impingement syndrome
- ▶ Rate of scapulothoracic asymmetry or increased topography with dynamic evaluation
  - ▷ 18% of asymptomatic individuals
  - ▷ 64% of patients with shoulder instability
  - ▷ 100% of patients with impingement syndrome

Conclusions

- ▶ Axioscapular muscle dysfunction is common in patients with instability and instability.
- ▶ Rehabilitation programs should address strengthening of both the serratus anterior and trapezius.

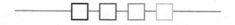

FEATURED ARTICLE

Authors: Itoi E, Kuechle DK, Newman SR, Morrey BF, An KN.

Title: Stabilising function of the biceps in stable and unstable shoulders.

Journal Information: *J Bone Joint Surg Br.* 1993;75:546–550.

Study Design: Cadaveric Study

- ▶ The purpose of this study was to determine the contributions of the long and short heads of the biceps to anterior stability of the shoulder joint with varying degrees of shoulder instability.
- ▶ 13 cadaveric shoulders studied
- ▶ The long head and short head of the biceps were replaced by spring devices.
- ▶ Humeral head position monitored by an electromagnetic tracking device with or without an anterior translational force

▸ Translation testing was performed by applying a 1.5-kg anterior force with the shoulder in 90 degrees of abduction.

▸ Loads of 0, 1.5, or 3 kg were applied to either the long head or short head of the biceps tendon in 60, 90, or 120 degrees of external rotation.

▸ Study performed with the capsule intact, vented, or damaged by a Bankart lesion

Results

▸ Anterior displacement of the humeral head was significantly decreased by loading both the long head and short head of the biceps in all capsular conditions when the arm was in 60 or 90 degrees of external rotation.

▸ At 120 degrees of external rotation, anterior displacement was significantly decreased by the long head and short head of the biceps loading only when there was a Bankart lesion.

Conclusions

▸ The long head and short head of the biceps have similar functions as anterior stabilizers of the shoulder joint with the arm in abduction and external rotation.

▸ Their stabilizing role increases as shoulder stability decreases.

▸ Since both heads of the biceps have a stabilizing function in resisting anterior head displacement, biceps strengthening should be part of the rehabilitation program in patients with chronic anterior shoulder instability.

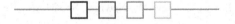

REVIEW ARTICLE

Wright RW, Baumgarten KM. Shoulder outcomes measures. *J Am Acad Orthop Surg*. 2010;18:436–444.

□ □ □ □

Shoulder Instability

Chapter **17**

FEATURE ARTICLE
Author: Blundell Bankart AS.
Title: The pathology and treatment of recurrent shoulder dislocation of the shoulder-joint.
Journal Information: *Br J Surg.* 1938;26:23–29.

Study Design: Cohort Study

▸ Historical description of Bankart's surgical technique to repair the essential anatomic defect in recurrent shoulder dislocation

▸ Bankart states that the typical lesion of recurrent shoulder dislocation is detachment of the glenoid ligament from the anterior margin of the glenoid.

▸ Bankart describes the dislocation mechanism leading to recurrent instability.

  ▷ Caused, not by a fall on the abducted arm, but by a fall either directly on the back of the shoulder or on the elbow

  ▷ The head of the humerus is forced out of the joint, not by leverage, but by a direct posterior-to-anterior force that shears off the fibrous capsule of the joint from its attachment to the fibrocartilaginous glenoid ligament.

  ▷ Because there is no tendency for the detached capsule to heal to the fibrocartilage, the defect is permanent and the humeral head is free to move forward over the anterior rim of the glenoid cavity with the slightest provocation.

Miller MD, Mauffrey C, Hak DJ.
Rapid Reference Review in Sports Medicine:
Pivotal Papers Revealed (pp 195-207).
© 2016 Taylor & Francis Group.

▶ The author reviews 4 other types of operations proposed for the management of recurrent shoulder dislocation, noting that they are either based on erroneous ideas of the pathology of recurrent shoulder dislocation or they ignore the pathology and attempt to deal empirically with the resulting clinical condition.

  ▷ Operations designed to diminish the size of the capsule

    » Bankart points out that the capsule in these cases is not unduly lax.

  ▷ Operations designed to give support to the capsule, particularly at its lowest part, where the dislocation is believed to take place during abduction of the arm

    » Bankart points out that the joint does not need support below, for it is not here that the dislocation takes place.

  ▷ Operations designed to hold the head of the humerus in place by means of an artificial ligament constructed either from the tendon of the long head of the biceps or from a free transplant of tendon or fascia

    » Bankart indicates that the unnatural tethering of the head of the humerus by an artificial ligament is a crude and irrational method of dealing with a straightforward anatomic defect.

  ▷ Operations that aim at the construction of a bony block in front of the head of the humerus

    » Bankart indicates that obstruction by means of an abnormal excrescence of bone is a crude and irrational method of dealing with a straightforward anatomic defect.

Results

▶ The author describes an operative experience of 27 consecutive cases of recurrent shoulder dislocation, all of which demonstrate the typical injury pattern of detachment of the glenoid ligament from the anterior margin of the glenoid.

▶ The surgical procedure reattaches the capsule to the anterior glenoid through a series of sutures passed through drill holes made in the anterior glenoid.

▶ All cases recovered full shoulder motion, and there were no reported recurrences.

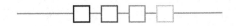

FEATURED ARTICLE

Authors: Rowe CR, Patel D, Southmayd WW.

Title: The Bankart procedure: a long-term end-result study.

Journal Information: *J Bone Joint Surg Am.* 1978;60:1–16.

A Top 100 Cited Articles in Clinical Orthopedic Sports Medicine

Study Design: Retrospective Review

- 161 patients (162 shoulders) operated on from 1946 to 1976 for recurrent anterior shoulder dislocation
- Surgical technique closely paralleled Bankart's original method
- Age range 15 to 47 years
- 145 available for follow-up
  - ▷ 124 were re-examined.
  - ▷ 21 answered a questionnaire.
- Operative findings
  - ▷ 85% had separation of the capsule from the anterior glenoid rim.
  - ▷ 77% had a Hill-Sachs lesion of the humeral head.
  - ▷ 73% had damage to the anterior glenoid rim (including fracture).
- Average follow-up 6 years
- Evaluation using a scoring system (0 to 100 points)
  - ▷ Stability (0 to 50 points)
  - ▷ Motion (0 to 20 points)
  - ▷ Function (0 to 30 points)

Results

- 3.5% (5/145) had a recurrent dislocation.
  - ▷ 2 were "loose jointed" and redislocation occurred by minimum trauma.
  - ▷ 3 redislocated as a result of major trauma.
- Rating at follow-up (by surgeon)
  - ▷ 74% excellent
  - ▷ 23% good
  - ▷ 3% poor

- Rating at follow-up (by patient)
  - ▷ 83% excellent
  - ▷ 15% good
  - ▷ 2% poor
- 69% of shoulders had full range of motion.
  - ▷ Only 2% of these shoulders redislocated.
- Glenoid rim fracture did not increase the risk of recurrence.
  - ▷ 2% (1/51) recurrence rate in patients with glenoid rim fractures
- Moderate to severe Hill-Sachs lesion only slightly increased the recurrence risk
  - ▷ No recurrences in 30 shoulders with mild Hill-Sachs lesion
  - ▷ 5% (4/80) recurrence rate shoulders with moderate to severe Hill-Sachs lesions
- 45/46 patients with dislocation on the dominant side returned to their preop competitive athletic activities.
- 30/31 patients with dislocations of the nondominant side returned to their preop competitive athletic activities.

Conclusions

- Post-op immobilization is not necessary following a Bankart repair if meticulous technique is used.
- Early return of motion and function can be expected.
- Resumption of athletic activities with no limitation of shoulder motion is possible for most patients.

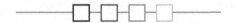

FEATURED ARTICLE

Authors: Andrews JR, Carson WG, McLeod WD.

Title: Glenoid labrum tears related to the long head of the biceps.

Journal Information: *Am J Sports Med.* 1985;13:337–341.

A Top 100 Cited Articles in Clinical Orthopedic Sports Medicine

Study Design: Retrospective Review

▶ Purpose: To describe a mechanism that might be responsible for tearing the glenoid labrum during throwing.

▶ This hypothesis is based on observations made during shoulder arthroscopy, 3D high-speed cinematography and computer-assisted analysis of the pitching mechanism, and biomechanical analysis of the biceps tendon during pitching.

▶ Retrospective review of 73 baseball pitchers and other throwing athletes who underwent arthroscopic examination of the dominant shoulder

▶ The relation of the long head of the biceps tendon to the superior portion of the glenoid labrum was observed arthroscopically during electrical stimulation of the biceps muscle.

▶ Average age 23 years

▶ Physical examination findings

▷ 79% with demonstrable popping or catching (especially with the arm in full abduction and full flexion close to the ear)

▷ 71% with tenderness

▷ 10% with anterior subluxation

▷ 8% with posterior subluxation

▷ 3% with multidirectional instability

▷ No patient demonstrated significant weakness of the rotator cuff or the biceps tendon.

Results

▶ All patients evaluated had some tearing of the glenoid labrum.

▶ 83% demonstrated tearing of the glenoid labrum in some portion of the anterosuperior region in the area of the biceps tendon/labrum complex.

▶ Tear location

▷ 60% (44 cases) anterosuperior

▷ 23% (17 cases) anterosuperior and posterosuperior

▷ 10% (7 cases) anterior

▷ 6% (4 cases) posterosuperior

▷ 1% (1 case) had an anterior bucket-handle tear.

▶ Other pathology

▷ 10% with partial biceps tendon tear near its origin

▷ 45% with supraspinatus tearing

▷ 73% (25/35) of baseball pitchers had partial tearing of the rotator cuff and 20% (7/35) had partial tearing of the long head of the biceps tendon.

- The long head of the biceps tendon appeared to originate through and be continuous with the superior portion of the glenoid labrum, and in many cases it appeared to have pulled the anterosuperior portion of the labrum off the glenoid.
- With electrical stimulation of the biceps muscle, the tendinous portion became quite taut, particularly near its attachment to the glenoid labrum, and actually lifted the labrum off the glenoid.
- Three-dimensional high-speed cinematography with computer analysis showed that the moment acting about the elbow joint to extend the joint through an arc of about 50 degrees was in excess of 600 inch-pounds.
- The extremely high velocity of elbow extension must be decelerated through the final 30 degrees of elbow extension.
- Only one muscle (biceps brachii) that provides the large deceleration forces in the follow-through phase of throwing traverses both the elbow and shoulder joints.
- Additional forces are generated in the biceps tendon in its function as a "shunt" muscle to stabilize the glenohumeral joint during throwing.

Conclusions

- The biceps tendon is subjected to large forces during throwing.
- Most tears of the glenoid labrum occur at the anterosuperior portion near the origin of the biceps tendon.
- The biceps tendon lifts the labrum off the glenoid when its muscle is stimulated.
- The authors therefore concluded that the long head of the biceps tendon might be a cause of tearing of the glenoid labrum in the throwing athlete.

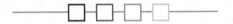

FEATURED ARTICLE

Authors: Morgan CD, Burkhart SS, Palmeri M, Gillespie M.

Title: Type II SLAP lesions: three subtypes and their relationships to superior instability and rotator cuff tears.

Journal Information: *Arthroscopy.* 1998;14:553–565.

A Top 100 Cited Articles in Clinical Orthopedic Sports Medicine

Study Design: Retrospective Review

▸ 102 type II superior labral tear from anterior to posterior (SLAP) lesions without associated anterior instability, Bankart lesion, or anterior inferior labral pathology

▸ All treated arthroscopically

Results

▸ Identified 3 distinct subtypes based on anatomic location
  ▷ 37% anterior
  ▷ 31% posterior
  ▷ 31% combined anterior and posterior

▸ Preop Speed and O'Brien tests were useful in predicting anterior lesions.

▸ Preop Jobe relocation test was useful in predicting posterior lesions.

▸ Rotator cuff tears were present in 31% of patients and were found to be lesion location specific.

▸ In posterior and combined anterior-posterior lesions, a drive-through sign was always present (despite absence of anterior-inferior labral pathology or a Bankart lesion) and was eliminated by repair of the posterior component of the SLAP lesion.

Conclusions

▸ Superior labral tear from anterior to posterior lesions with a posterior component develop posterior-superior instability that manifests itself by a secondary anterior-inferior pseudolaxity (drive-through sign).

▸ Chronic superior instability leads to secondary lesion-location–specific rotator cuff tears that begin as partial-thickness tears from inside the joint.

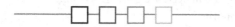

FEATURED ARTICLE

Authors: Bottoni CR, Wilckens JH, DeBerardino TM, D'Alleyrand JC, Rooney RC, Harpstrite JK, Arciero RA.

Title: A prospective, randomized evaluation of arthroscopic stabilization versus nonoperative treatment in patients with acute, traumatic, first-time shoulder dislocations.

Journal Information: *Am J Sports Med.* 2002;30:576–580.

Study Design: Prospective Randomized Study

▶ Young, male, active-duty personnel with acute traumatic shoulder dislocations randomized to:

  ▷ Nonoperative treatment (14 patients)

  ▷ Arthroscopic Bankart repair (10 patients)

▶ Both groups immobilized for 4 weeks, followed by a supervised rehabilitation program

▶ Average age 22.4 years (18 to 26 years), all men

▶ Average follow-up 36 months

▶ 3 patients lost to follow-up

▶ Outcome assessments

  ▷ Single assessment numeric evaluation (SANE)

  ▷ L'Insalata shoulder evaluation (addresses the use of the shoulder for both daily activities and sports)

  ▷ Shoulder range of motion

  ▷ Recurrent instability

Results

▶ 75% (9/12) of patients in nonoperative treatment group developed recurrent instability.

  ▷ 6/9 required subsequent open Bankart repair.

▶ 11.1% (1/9) of patients in the arthroscopic Bankart repair group developed recurrent instability.

▶ No statistical difference in shoulder range of motion between the 2 groups

▶ Average SANE

  ▷ 57 (46 to 98) in nonoperative group

  ▷ 88 (60 to 100) in operative group ($P < 0.002$)

▶ Average L'Insalata score

  ▷ 73 (46 to 92) in nonoperative group

  ▷ 94 (65 to 98) in operative group ($P < 0.002$)

Conclusions

▶ Arthroscopic stabilization of traumatic, first-time anterior shoulder dislocations significantly reduces the recurrence rate and improves outcomes in young athletes.

▶ Restoration of the capsulolabral complex to its anatomic position can lead to normal function without instability.

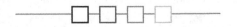

FEATURED ARTICLE

Authors: Burkhead WZ, Rockwood CA.

Title: Treatment of instability of the shoulder with an exercise program.

Journal Information: *JBJS Am.* 1992;74:890–896.

Study Design: Retrospective Review

▶ Purpose: To report on the effect of a specific rehab program for patients with traumatic or atraumatic multidirectional shoulder instability

▶ 140 shoulders in 115 patients with traumatic or atraumatic recurrent anterior, posterior, or multidirectional subluxation

▶ All treated with a specific set of muscle-strengthening exercises

▶ Average follow-up 46 months (2 to 6 years)

▶ Grading system
   ▷ Function (0 to 50 points)
   ▷ Pain (0 to 10 points)
   ▷ Stability (0 to 30 points)
   ▷ Motion (0 to 10 points)
   ▷ Excellent (90 to 100 points)
   ▷ Good (70 to 89 points)
   ▷ Fair (40 to 69 points)
   ▷ Poor (≤ 39 points)

Results

▶ Only 16% (12/74 shoulders) who had a traumatic subluxation had a good or excellent result.
   ▷ 18% (6/24 shoulders) with a first-time traumatic anterior dislocation had a good or excellent result.
   ▷ 33% (2/6 shoulders) with a first-time traumatic posterior dislocation had a good or excellent result.
   ▷ 9% (3/34 shoulders) with a history of a prior dislocation had a good or excellent result.

▶ 80% (53/66 shoulders) who had an atraumatic subluxation had a good or excellent result.
   ▷ 2/5 patients with associated psychological problems responded well to the therapy program

▷ 87.5% (14/16 shoulders) categorized as voluntary subluxation but without psychological problems had good or excellent results

▷ 87% (39/45 shoulders) categorized as involuntary subluxation had good or excellent results

Conclusion

▸ Significant effort must be made to identify the etiology of the instability through history, physical examination, and radiographs.

▸ Conservative therapy is best suited for patients with an atraumatic etiology for their shoulder instability.

▸ The authors recommend a trial of specific resistance-strengthening exercises for patients with atraumatic and multidirectional shoulder instability before reconstructive surgery is considered.

▷ There is a high rate of complications associated with shoulder reconstructive procedures.

▷ There is a high rate of success with rehabilitation exercises for this group of patients.

▸ The authors recommended that once a stable shoulder has developed that the exercises still be done at least 2 to 3 times per week since some patients developed recurrent symptoms when they stopped the exercises.

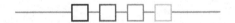

CLASSIC ARTICLE

Authors: Neer CS 2nd, Foster CR.

Title: Inferior capsular shift for involuntary inferior and multidirectional instability of the shoulder: a preliminary report.

Journal Information: *J Bone Joint Surg Am.* 1980;62:897–908.

A Top 100 Cited Articles in Clinical Orthopedic Sports Medicine

---

Study Design: Retrospective Review

▸ 36 patients with involuntary inferior and multidirectional instability of the shoulder

▸ Average age 24 years (range 15 to 55 years), 18 men, 18 women

- Generalized hyperlaxity of joints seen in 17 patients
- The interval from the onset of shoulder disability to operation averaged 3 years (range 1 to 21 years)
- All were treated with an inferior capsular shift (40 shoulders in 36 patients).
  - ▷ A flap of the capsule, reinforced by overlying tendon, is shifted to reduce capsular and ligamentous redundancy on all 3 sides.
  - ▷ Offers the advantage of correcting multidirectional instability through one incision without damage to the articular surface
  - ▷ Performed through either an anterior or posterior surgical approach
- Outcome graded as satisfactory or unsatisfactory
  - ▷ Satisfactory = no recurrence of dislocation or subluxation, no significant pain, full activities, normal strength, and within 10 degrees of full elevation and 40 degrees of rotation compared with the contralateral shoulder
  - ▷ Unsatisfactory = failure to meet aforementioned criteria
- Since the contralateral shoulder was usually hypermobile, 20 degrees less rotation was considered ideal for the repaired shoulder.
- 32 shoulders were followed for more than 1 year; 17 shoulders were followed for more than 2 years.

Results

- 1 shoulder began subluxating again within 7 months after operation. Failure was thought to be due to a Bankart lesion of the anterior glenoid labrum that was not repaired.
- 1 other patient who had been followed for 4 years had 2 episodes of disabling pain 2 years apart. No redislocation occurred, and the pain abated with rest followed by exercises.
- Neurapraxia of the axillary nerve occurred in 3 patients, a reminder that this procedure places the axillary nerve in jeopardy.
- Identified 4 aspects that should be considered in the evaluation of patients with inferior and multidirectional shoulder instability.
  1. It is important to exclude voluntary dislocators, as they may willfully cause an operative procedure to fail.
  2. Inferior instability is not always symptomatic, and it may be that another local lesion is causing the pain.
  3. Mildly symptomatic inferior instability can at times be controlled by altering patient activity and with specific muscle exercises. Surgery should not be considered until efforts to strengthen the rotator cuff muscles and deltoid have failed.
  4. Accurate assessment of the direction of instability is essential in planning the operative repair.

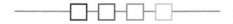

FEATURED REVIEW ARTICLE

Authors: Matsen FA, Harryman DT, Sidles JA.

Title: Mechanics of glenohumeral instability.

Journal Information: *Clin Sports Med.* 1991;10:783–788.

▸ This article is designed as a practical guide to understanding the mechanism, diagnosis, and management of glenohumeral instability.
▸ Emphasizes the authors' experience that treatment needs to be based on the history and physical examination
▸ Imaging tests, examination under anesthesia, or arthroscopic findings rarely modify the planned treatment that is based on history and physical examination.

Results

▸ Outlines types of instability
  ▷ TUBS
    » **T**raumatic event results in **U**nidirectional anterior instability with a **B**ankart lesion, and **S**urgery is usually required to regain stability
    » "Torn loose"
  ▷ AMBRII
    » **A**traumatic onset of **M**ultidirectional instability that is accompanied by **B**ilateral laxity and **R**ehabilitation is usually required to regain stability
    » If surgery is required, a global capsulorraphy with tightening of the **I**nferior capsule and the rotator **I**nterval
    » "Born loose"

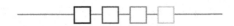

REVIEW ARTICLES

Gaskill TR, Taylor, DC, Millett PJ. Management of multidirectional instability of the shoulder. *J Am Acad Orthop Surg.* 2011;19:758–767.

Millett PJ, Clavert P, Hatch III CFR, Warner JJP. Recurrent posterior shoulder instability. *J Am Acad Orthop Surg.* 2006;14:464–476.

Harris JD, Romeo AA. Arthroscopic management of the contact athlete with instability. *Clin Sports Med.* 2013;32:709–730.

Shoulder Dislocation

Chapter **18**

FEATURED ARTICLE

Authors: Hovelius L, Augustini BG, Fredin H, Johansson O, Norlin R, Thorling J.

Title: Primary anterior shoulder dislocation of the shoulder in young patients. A ten-year prospective study.

Journal Information: *J Bone Joint Surg.* 1996;78A:1677–1684.

A Top 100 Cited Articles in Clinical Orthopedic Sports Medicine

Study Design: Prospective Randomized Study

▶ Prospective multicenter study of 245 patients who had had 247 primary anterior shoulder dislocations assigned to 1 of 3 treatments:

  ▷ Immobilization with the arm tied with a bandage to the torso for 3 to 4 weeks after reduction of the dislocation

  ▷ Use of a sling, which was discontinued after the patient was comfortable

  ▷ Immobilization for various durations

▶ Patients followed for 10 years at 27 Swedish hospitals

▶ Age at time of the dislocation 12 to 40 years

Results at 10 Years

▶ 129 shoulders (52%) had no additional dislocation.

▶ 116 shoulders (48%) had a recurrent dislocation.

Miller MD, Mauffrey C, Hak DJ.
Rapid Reference Review in Sports Medicine:
Pivotal Papers Revealed (pp 209-213).
© 2016 Taylor & Francis Group.

- 58 shoulders (23%) had a recurrent dislocation necessitating operative treatment.
  - ▷ Recurrent dislocation necessitating operative treatment occurred in:
  - ▷ 34% of patients ages 12 to 22
  - ▷ 28% of patients ages 23 to 29
  - ▷ 9% of patients ages 30 to 40
- 24 shoulders with at least 2 recurrent dislocations during the first 2 to 5 years seemed to have stabilized spontaneously without operative intervention.
- Dislocation of the contralateral shoulder occurred in 31 patients.
  - ▷ Contralateral dislocation occurred in:
  - ▷ 16% of patients ages 12 to 22
  - ▷ 21% of patients ages 23 to 29
  - ▷ 3% of patients ages 30 to 40
- The type and duration of initial treatment had no effect on rate of recurrent dislocation.
- There were radiographs of 185 shoulders at the time of the primary dislocation.
  - ▷ 99 shoulders (54%) showed a Hill-Sachs lesion.
  - ▷ Presence of a Hill-Sachs lesion was associated with a significantly worse prognosis with regard to recurrence ($P < 0.04$).
- Radiographs of 208 shoulders at the 10-year follow-up examination
  - ▷ 23 shoulders (11%) had mild arthropathy
  - ▷ 18 shoulders (9%) had moderate or severe arthropathy
  - ▷ Some of the shoulders that had arthropathy had no recurrence.

Conclusions

- Risk of recurrent dislocation is higher in younger patients.
- Authors reported that the prognosis after a primary glenohumeral dislocation, even in younger patients, was not as devastating as had previously been reported.
- Some shoulders with recurrent dislocation become stable over time.
- A shorter 3- to 4-week period of immobilization after reduction of the primary dislocation did not appear to adversely affect patient outcome.

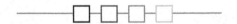

CLASSIC ARTICLE

Author: Rowe CR.

Title: Prognosis in dislocations of the shoulder.

Journal Information: *J Bone Joint Surg Am.* 1956;38-A:957–977.

Study Design: Retrospective Review

▶ 500 shoulder dislocations in a series of 488 patients treated over 20 years
▶ Follow-up available on 313 shoulders (63%)
▶ Mean follow-up 4.8 years

Results

▶ Characteristics of dislocations
  ▷ 2% of dislocations were posterior.
  ▷ 2.4% of patients sustained bilateral dislocations.
  ▷ 2% of patients sustaining a dislocation had epilepsy.
  ▷ 5.4% incidence of associated nerve injury
  ▷ 24% had an associated fracture of the shoulder girdle.
  ▷ 15% had an associated greater tuberosity fracture.
▶ Primary shoulder dislocations occurred as frequently in patients > 45 years as in patients < 45 years of age.
▶ 38% rate of redislocation
▶ Incidence of recurrent shoulder dislocation was very high in the second decade (92% incidence), but showed marked decrease after age 50 (12% incidence).
▶ Patient age at the time of the primary shoulder dislocation was the most significant single prognostic factor
▶ Patients who did not redislocate had a higher average age.
▶ Usually greater initial injury force was associated with a lower incidence of redislocation.
▶ Humeral-head defects were seen in 38% of the primary dislocations and in 57% of recurrent dislocations.
▶ Humeral-head defects were associated with an increase in the incidence of redislocation (82%).

- Incidence of redislocation was not very much affected by the type and length of shoulder immobilization following dislocation.
  - ▷ Although there was a high incidence of redislocation in patients who were not immobilized or who were immobilized for only a very short period, longer periods of immobilization were not associated with a significant decrease in redislocation.
- 70% of redislocations following the primary dislocation occurred within the first 2 years.
- 52% redislocation rate within 2 years in patients who underwent surgical treatment for recurrent dislocation.

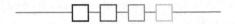

FEATURED ARTICLE

Authors: Baker CL Jr, Uribe JW, Whitman C.

Title: Arthroscopic evaluation of acute initial shoulder dislocations.

Journal Information: *Am J Sports Med.* 1990;18:25–28.

Study Design: Retrospective Review

- 45 shoulders that were evaluated arthroscopically within 10 days of dislocation
  - ▷ No prior history of shoulder problems
  - ▷ Age < 30 years
  - ▷ Dislocation confirmed by radiograph or reduction by a physician
- Identified and classified the associated pathoanatomy following initial traumatic shoulder dislocation
- Average age 21.2 years (14 to 28 years), 42 men, 3 women
- Authors present a classification of the lesions found in acute shoulder dislocations

Results

- Group 1 (6 shoulders): Capsular tears with no labral lesions, stable under anesthesia, and had no or minimal hemarthrosis
- Group 2 (11 shoulders): Capsular tears and partial labral detachments, mildly unstable, and had mild to moderate hemarthrosis

▶ Group 3 (28 shoulders): Capsular tears with complete labral detachments, grossly unstable, and had large hemarthrosis

Conclusions

▶ Authors concluded that the age of the patient at the time of initial dislocation, the force of dislocation, and the type of initial traumatic lesion combine to predispose the shoulder to recurrent dislocation.

▶ Arthroscopy performed after the initial traumatic episode of dislocation may, therefore, be beneficial in determining which patients are prone to recurrent dislocation and adjust their treatment regimen appropriately.

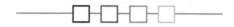

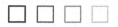

Impingement Syndrome

Chapter 19

FEATURED ARTICLE

Authors: Flatow EL, Soslowsky LJ, Ticker JB, Pawluk RJ, Hepler M, Ark J, Mow VC, Bigliani LU.

Title: Excursion of the rotator cuff under the acromion: patterns of subacromial contact.

Journal Information: *Am J Sports Med.* 1994; 22:779–788.

Study Design: Cadaveric Study

▶ The bursa and supraspinatus insertion on the greater tuberosity must repeatedly pass beneath the acromion with the arm in varying degrees of elevation and rotation during forceful overhead activity.

▶ There is little or no quantitative data concerning normal patterns of contact between the acromion and the underlying cuff tissues and greater tuberosity or abnormal contact patterns created by impingement.

▶ 9 fresh-frozen human cadaveric shoulders

▶ Shoulders were elevated in the scapular plane in 2 different humeral rotations by applying forces along action lines of the rotator cuff and deltoid muscles.

▶ An optical stereophotogrammetry technique was used to determine the contact areas at the subacromial articulation.

▶ Radiographs measured acromiohumeral interval and position of greater tuberosity

Miller MD, Mauffrey C, Hak DJ.
*Rapid Reference Review in Sports Medicine:
Pivotal Papers Revealed (pp 215-223).*
© 2016 Taylor & Francis Group.

Results

▸ Contact starts at the anterolateral edge of the acromion at 0 degrees of elevation.

▸ Contact shifts medially with arm elevation.

▸ On the humeral surface, contact shifts from proximal to distal on the supraspinatus tendon with arm elevation.

▸ When external rotation is decreased, there are distal and posterior shifts in contact.

▸ Acromial undersurface and rotator cuff tendons are in closest proximity between 60 and 120 degrees of elevation.

▸ Contact was consistently more pronounced for type III acromions.

▸ Mean acromiohumeral interval was 11.1 mm at 0 degrees of elevation and decreased to 5.7 mm at 90 degrees when greater tuberosity was closest to the acromion

Conclusions

▸ Contact centers on the supraspinatus insertion, suggesting altered excursion of the greater tuberosity may initially damage this rotator cuff region.

▸ Conditions limiting external rotation or elevation may also increase rotator cuff compression.

▸ Marked increase in contact with type III acromions supports the role of anterior acromioplasty when clinically indicated, usually in older patients with primary impingement.

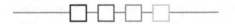

FEATURED ARTICLE

Authors: Spangehl MJ, Hawkins RH, McCormack RG, Loomer RL.

Title: Arthroscopic versus open acromioplasty: a prospective randomized blinded study.

Journal Information: *J Shoulder Elbow Surg.* 2002;11:101–108.

Study Design: Prospective Randomized Study

- ▶ Purpose: To determine whether arthroscopic acromioplasty is equivalent or superior to open acromioplasty
- ▶ Prospective, randomized, controlled, blinded clinical trial
- ▶ 71 patients with a clinical diagnosis of impingement syndrome randomized to:
  - ▷ Arthroscopic acromioplasty
  - ▷ Open acromioplasty
  - ▷ Randomization stratified for age > 50, associated ligamentous laxity, and presence of an ongoing compensation claim
  - ▷ Groups very similar with regard to duration of symptoms, shoulder functional demands, age, sex, hand dominance, mechanism of onset, range of motion, strength, joint laxity, and presence of a compensation claim
- ▶ 9 patients were excluded after randomization due to presence of a full-thickness rotator cuff tear
- ▶ 62 patients completed study
- ▶ Average age 41 years, 49 men, 13 women
- ▶ Average follow-up 25 months, minimum 12 months
- ▶ Outcome measurements
  - ▷ Visual analog scale for pain
  - ▷ Visual analog scale for function
  - ▷ University of California, Los Angeles (UCLA) shoulder scores
  - ▷ Visual analog scales for post-op improvement, patient satisfaction, and a variety of clinical measures
- ▶ An independent blinded examiner assessed all patients.

Results

- ▶ No significant difference between groups in visual analog scales for:
  - ▷ Post-op improvement ($P = 0.30$)
  - ▷ Patient satisfaction ($P = 0.94$)
  - ▷ UCLA shoulder score ($P = 0.69$)
  - ▷ Strength ($P = 0.62$)
- ▶ Open acromioplasty was superior to arthroscopic acromioplasty for:
  - ▷ Pain ($P = 0.01$)
  - ▷ Function ($P = 0.01$)
- ▶ Overall, 67% of patients had a good or excellent result.
- ▶ 87% of patients without ongoing compensation claims had or good or excellent result
- ▶ Repeat (open) acromioplasty was performed in 5 patients in the unsuccessful arthroscopic group without improvement

Conclusions

▸ Both open and arthroscopic acromioplasty provided significant relief for impingement syndrome symptoms in patients with an intact rotator cuff.

▸ Open technique yielded better pain relief and functional improvement

▸ In terms of subjective improvement, overall satisfaction, UCLA score, and shoulder strength, the 2 techniques were equivalent.

▸ Unsettled compensation is a predictor of poor outcome.

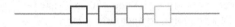

FEATURED ARTICLE

Authors: Neer CS, Marberry TA.

Title: *On the disadvantages of radical acromionectomy.*

Journal Information: *J Bone Joint Surg Am.* 1981;63:416–419.

Study Design: Retrospective Review

▸ 30 consecutive patients who previously had a radical acromionectomy (≥ 80% of acromion resected) performed elsewhere

▸ Surgical indication cited for the radical acromionectomy
  ▹ 18 rotator cuff tear
  ▹ 7 malunited fractures of the proximal end of the humerus or of the greater tuberosity
  ▹ 5 various diagnoses (bursitis, rheumatoid arthritis, or failed surgery)

▸ Average age 56 years (35 to 81), 17 women, 13 men

Results

▸ All patients undergoing radical acromionectomy had poor results.

▸ 27 had persistent pain.

▸ All had marked shoulder weakness.

▸ None could raise the arm above the horizontal.

▸ 8 had serious wound complications.

▸ All objected to the appearance of the shoulder.

Conclusions

▶ Radical acromionectomy weakens the deltoid muscle in 2 ways:

▷ Removing the fulcrum afforded by the acromion to the deltoid for its function of shoulder abduction and elevation

▷ By retraction of the middle section of the deltoid muscle, which became adherent to either the rotator cuff on the humerus or both and soon became fibrotic and permanently shortened

▶ Weakening of the deltoid in patients with rotator cuff tears made the shoulder even more disabled.

▶ Patients with pain from a retracted greater tuberosity after a fracture were not relieved by acromionectomy because the tuberosity continued to impinge against the glenoid.

▶ Patients with rheumatoid shoulders were not relieved by acromionectomy because of persistent pain due to involvement of the joint surface and subdeltoid adhesions.

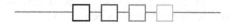

FEATURED ARTICLE

Authors: Morrison DS, Frogameni AD, Woodworth P.

Title: Non-operative treatment of subacromial impingement syndrome.

Journal Information: *J Bone Joint Surg Am.* 1997;79:732–737.

Study Design: Retrospective Review

▶ 616 patients (636 shoulders) with subacromial impingement syndrome treated nonoperatively

▶ All patients had a positive impingement sign and absence of other shoulder abnormalities of the shoulder (no full-thickness rotator cuff tears, acromioclavicular joint osteoarthrosis, instability, or adhesive capsulitis).

▶ Treatment

▷ Anti-inflammatory medication (indomethacin 150 mg daily in divided doses × 3 weeks)

▷ A specific, supervised physical therapy regimen consisting of isotonic exercises for rotator cuff strengthening

- ▶ Average age 42 years (15 to 81 years), 386 men, 230 women
- ▶ Average follow-up 27 months (6 to 81 months)
- ▶ Outcome assessment
  - ▷ Questioned regarding pain, shoulder function, work status, recurrence of symptoms, and overall satisfaction
  - ▷ UCLA shoulder rating scale
    - » 35-point scale that combines scores for pain, function, the range of active forward elevation, strength in forward elevation, and patient satisfaction

Results

- ▶ 67% (413 patients) satisfactory result
- ▶ 28% (172 patients) no improvement and went on to arthroscopic subacromial decompression
- ▶ 5% (31 patients) had an unsatisfactory result but declined additional treatment.
- ▶ 18% (74 patients) of the 413 patients with successful results had a symptomatic recurrence during the follow-up period, but these symptoms resolved with rest or with resumption of the exercise program.
- ▶ Outcome with respect to age
  - ▷ Patients > 60 years had the poorest results.
  - ▷ Patients ≤20 and patients 41 to 60 years old did better than those who were 21 to 40 years old.
- ▶ Outcome with respect to duration of symptoms
  - ▷ 78% of patients with symptoms < 4 weeks had a satisfactory result.
  - ▷ 63% of patients with symptoms from 1 to 6 months had a satisfactory result.
  - ▷ 67% of patients with symptoms > 6 months had a satisfactory result.
- ▶ Outcome with respect to acromial morphology
  - ▷ 91% of patients with a type I acromion had a successful result.
  - ▷ 68% of patients with a type II acromion had a satisfactory result.
  - ▷ 64% of patients with a type III acromion had a satisfactory result.
- ▶ Shoulder dominance, gender, and concomitant acromioclavicular joint tenderness did not significantly affect the result.

Conclusions

- ▶ Goals of nonoperative subacromial impingement syndrome treatment are:
  - ▷ Decrease subacromial inflammation
  - ▷ Allow healing of the compromised rotator cuff
  - ▷ Restore satisfactory function to the painful shoulder

- Nonoperative management was successful in the majority (67%) of patients.
- Investigators found that patients with a type Ill acromion fared no worse than those who had a type II acromion, and suggested that perhaps there is a nonanatomic mechanism for rotator cuff pain in addition to impingement.
- Poorer results may be expected in patients > 60 years old because of the presence of undiagnosed full-thickness rotator cuff tears.
- It is unclear why the patients 21 to 40 years old had less satisfactory results in this study.

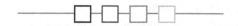

CLASSIC ARTICLE

Author: Neer CS II.

Title: Anterior acromioplasty for chronic impingement syndrome in the shoulder: a preliminary report.

Journal Information: *J Bone Joint Surg Am*. 1972;54:41–50.

A Top 100 Cited Articles in Clinical Orthopedic Sports Medicine

---

Study Design: Retrospective Review

- 50 shoulders in 46 patients with mechanical impingement who underwent open anterior acromioplasty between 1965 and 1970
- Average age 51.5 years (range 42 to 73 years), 28 men, 18 women
- Supraspinatus pathology found at surgery
  - ▷ Tendonitis or partial tear: 19 shoulders
  - ▷ Full-thickness tear: 20 shoulders
  - ▷ Evidence of residual impingement after prior lateral acromionectomy: 11 shoulders
- Average follow-up 2.5 years (range 9 months to 5 years)
  - ▷ Follow-up available for 47 shoulders
  - ▷ 29 by examination
  - ▷ 18 by questionnaire

- Also dissected 100 scapulae and identified a characteristic proliferative spur and ridge on the anterior lip and undersurface of the anterior process of the acromion in 11 specimens

Results

- Graded as:
  - ▷ Satisfactory
    - » Patient was satisfied with the operation.
    - » No significant pain
    - » Full use of the shoulder
    - » < 20 degrees of limitation of overhead extension
    - » At least 75% of normal strength
  - ▷ Unsatisfactory
    - » Failure to meet the aforementioned criteria
- No deep infections
- 5 subcutaneous hematomas that spontaneously resolved
- 16 patients with chronic bursitis with fraying or partial supraspinatus tear
  - ▷ 15 satisfactory
  - ▷ 1 unsatisfactory
  - ▷ 3 shoulders not evaluated
- 20 patients with full-thickness supraspinatus tears
  - ▷ 19 satisfactory
  - ▷ 1 unsatisfactory
- 11 patients that had undergone prior lateral acromionectomy
  - ▷ 4 satisfactory
  - ▷ 7 unsatisfactory

Conclusions

- Anterior acromioplasty may offer better relief of chronic pain in selected patients with mechanical impingement.
- It provides better exposure for repairing tears of the supraspinatus.
- It may prevent further impingement and wear at the critical area without loss of deltoid power.

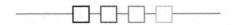

REVIEW ARTICLES

Harrison AK, Flatow EL. Subacromial impingement syndrome. *J Am Acad Orthop Surg.* 2011;19:701–708.

Hawkins RJ, Kennedy JC. Impingement syndrome in athletes. *Am J Sports Med.* 1980;8:151–158. (*A Top 100 Cited Articles in Clinical Orthopedic Sports Medicine*)

Rotator Cuff Tears

Chapter **20**

> ### FEATURED ARTICLE
>
> **Authors:** Gartsman GM, Khan M, Hammerman SM.
>
> **Title:** Arthroscopic repair of full-thickness tears of the rotator cuff.
>
> **Journal Information:** *J Bone Joint Surg Am.* 1998;80:832–840.

Study Design: Retrospective Review

- 73 patients who underwent arthroscopic repair of full-thickness rotator cuff tears
- Average age 60.7 years (31 to 82 years), 39 men, 34 women
- Average follow-up 30 months (24 to 40 months)
- Outcome measurements
  - ▷ University of California, Los Angeles (UCLA) shoulder score
  - ▷ American Shoulder and Elbow Surgeons (ASES) rating scale
  - ▷ Constant score
  - ▷ SF-36
  - ▷ Visual analog scale (VAS) for pain
- Tear size
  - ▷ Average tear length 12 mm, average tear width 27 mm
  - ▷ 11 small (< 1 cm)
  - ▷ 45 medium (1 to 3 cm)

Miller MD, Mauffrey C, Hak DJ.
Rapid Reference Review in Sports Medicine:
Pivotal Papers Revealed (pp 225-248).
© 2016 Taylor & Francis Group.

▷ 11 large (< 3 to 5 cm)

▷ 6 massive (> 5 cm)

▶ Tendon repair

▷ 69 tendons repaired anatomically

▷ 4 tendons repaired an average 3 mm (2 to 8 mm) medial to the anatomic tendon insertion site

▷ Average of 2.3 (1 to 4) suture anchors used

Results

▶ Active and passive ranges of motion improved significantly after the procedure ($P = 0.0001$)

▶ Strength of resisted elevation improved from 7.5 to 14.0 pounds ($P = 0.0001$)

▶ Average total UCLA score improved from 12.4 to 31.1 points ($P = 0.0001$)

▷ Average UCLA pain component improved from 2.4 to 8.6 points

▶ Average total ASES score improved from 30.7 to 87.6 points ($P = 0.0001$)

▶ Average Constant score improved from 41.7 to 83.6 points ($P = 0.0001$)

▶ 78% (57 patients) rated their pain relief as good or excellent on VAS.

▶ 90% (66 patients) rated their satisfaction as good or excellent.

▶ None of the shoulders were rated as good or excellent before the operation.

▶ 84% (61 shoulders) were rated as good or excellent at most recent follow-up

▶ Significant improvements in SF-36 scales and summary measures ($P = 0.0015$)

Conclusions

▶ Arthroscopic repair of full-thickness tears of the rotator cuff produced good results for patient satisfaction, pain relief, and general health.

▶ Arthroscopic repair offers several advantages, including:

▷ Smaller incisions

▷ Access to the glenohumeral joint for the inspection and treatment of intra-articular lesions

▷ No need for deltoid detachment

▷ Less soft tissue dissection

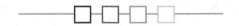

FEATURED ARTICLE

Authors: Sher JS, Uribe JW, Posada A, Murphy BJ, Zlatkin MB.

Title: Abnormal findings on magnetic resonance images of asymptomatic shoulders.

Journal Information: *J Bone Joint Surg Am.* 1995;77:10–15.

A Top 100 Cited Articles in Clinical Orthopedic Sports Medicine

Study Design: Cohort Study

▶ Evaluated shoulder magnetic resonance imaging (MRI) of 96 asymptomatic volunteers who were recruited for the study through local advertisement
▶ Average age 53 years (19 to 88 years), 47 men, 49 women
  ▷ Divided into 3 groups according to age:
    » 19 to 39 years (25 subjects)
    » 40 to 60 years (25 subjects)
    » Older than 60 years (46 subjects)
      ⟩ Subjects > 60 years were subjectively categorized on the basis of history of occupational and athletic involvement in over-the-head activities into:
        ⟩ Sedentary
        ⟩ Active
▶ Magnetic resonance imaging studies were reviewed independently by 2 diagnostic radiologists.

Results

▶ 34% (33/96) overall prevalence of rotator cuff tears in all age groups
  ▷ 14 full-thickness tears (15%)
  ▷ 19 partial-thickness tears (20%)
▶ Frequency of full-thickness tears increased significantly with age ($P < 0.001$).
▶ Frequency of partial-thickness tears also increased significantly with age ($P < 0.05$).
▶ 54% (25/46) of subjects > 60 years old had a rotator cuff tear.
  ▷ 28% (13/46) had a full-thickness tear.
  ▷ 26% (12/46) had a partial-thickness tear.
  ▷ No significant difference between the sedentary and active subgroups ($P = 0.16$)

- 28% (7/25) of subjects ages 40 to 60 had a rotator cuff tear.
  ▷ 4% (1/25) had a full-thickness rotator cuff tear.
  ▷ 24% (6/25) had a partial-thickness tear.
- 4% (1/25) of subjects ages 19 to 39 had a rotator cuff tear.
  ▷ No full-thickness rotator cuff tears
  ▷ 4% (1/25) had a partial-thickness tear.

Conclusions

- Magnetic resonance imaging identified a high prevalence of rotator cuff tears in asymptomatic individuals.
- Rotator cuff tears were increasingly frequent with advancing age and were compatible with normal, painless, functional activity.
- Magnetic resonance imaging findings alone cannot be used as a basis for determining the need for operative treatment; rather, they must be correlated with clinical findings.

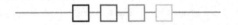

FEATURED ARTICLE

Authors: Hawkins RJ, Misamore GW, Hobeika PE.

Title: Surgery for full-thickness rotator-cuff tears.

Journal Information: *J Bone Joint Surg Am.* 1985;67:1349–1355.

Study Design: Retrospective Review

- 100 consecutive rotator cuff tears treated surgically between 1976 and 1981
- Average age 57.4 (26 to 76 years), 78 men, 22 women
- Average follow-up 4.2 years (2 to 7 years)
- 3 patients were lost to follow-up before the 2-year minimum.
- Since their policy was to treat acute tears conservatively, this series included only patients with a painful subacute or chronic rotator cuff tear.
- Operative exploration revealed
  ▷ 16 small tears (< 1 cm)
  ▷ 36 moderate size tears (1 to 3 cm)

▷ 21 large tears (3 to 5 cm)

▷ 27 massive tears (> 5 cm)

▶ Rotator cuff tear repair was achieved in 94 patients.

   ▷ 22 had direct end-to-end repair.

   ▷ 72 medial ends of the torn cuff were sutured to a trough in the humerus.

▶ Repair was not possible in 6 patients with massive tears, and these patients were treated with partial acromioplasty and debridement of the tendon ends and bursa.

▶ Assessment at follow-up

   ▷ Pain assessment (marked, moderate, only after stressful activity, slight, or none)

   ▷ Functional capabilities (unable, with aid, with difficulty, minimum compromise, or normal)

   ▷ Active and passive ranges of motion

   ▷ Strength grading

   ▷ Patient's subjective evaluation of post-op result (worse, same, moderately improved, or much improved)

Results

▶ 86 patients had slight or no pain post-op.

▶ All but 3 patients had some pain relief after the surgical treatment.

▶ Function of the shoulder was improved in most aspects in all but 8 patients.

▶ More than half of the patients continued to have weakness after surgery.

▶ Post-op active range of motion of the shoulder was directly proportional to size of the cuff tear.

▶ Tear size of did not significantly affect the results, although patients with a smaller tear tended to fare slightly better.

▶ There was a statistically significant difference in shoulder function between patients with a small tear compared to those with a massive tear ($P < 0.01$).

▶ There was a statistically significant difference in strength between patients with either a small or a moderate tear compared to those with a large or massive tear ($P < 0.05$).

▶ Only 2/14 Workers' Compensation Board patients who were not working preop returned to their jobs post-op.

▶ It took workers' compensation patients twice as long to return to work.

Conclusions

▶ Most patients had improved shoulder function, but the authors suspected that this improvement was primarily related to pain relief because there was only modest improvement in strength.

- Although many patients had either some residual pain or weakness or limitation of motion on follow-up, nearly all thought they were improved by surgery.
- Although the patients with the larger tears tended to have more severe symptoms and signs, the authors could not predict the tear size that was likely to be seen at surgery.
- The authors recommend operations for workers' compensation patients only for pain relief, making it clear that surgery probably will not enable the patient to return to work if he or she had not been working preop.

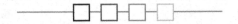

FEATURED ARTICLE

Authors: Gerber C, Schneeberger AG, Beck M, Schlegel U.

Title: Mechanical strength of repairs of the rotator cuff.

Journal Information: *J Bone Joint Surg Br.* 1994;67:371–380.

Study Design: Biomechanical Study

- The purpose of this investigation was to study the mechanical properties of several current tendon-to-bone suture techniques used in rotator cuff repair.
- Examined frequently used sutures on an Instron universal testing machine
  ▷ Measured elongation under load
  ▷ Ultimate tensile strength
- Examined 8 different knot patterns (Figure 20-1)
- Then used the best-performing sutures (Ethibond 1 and 3 and Tevdek II 1, both braided polyester) to examine 9 different techniques of tendon grasping in sheep infraspinatus tendons (Figure 20-2)
- The more successful tendon-grasping techniques were retested with augmentation by 1.4-mm-thick, firm absorbable poly (L-/D-lactide) membrane.
- Studied the mechanical properties of several methods of anchorage to bone using osteoporotic cadaveric specimens

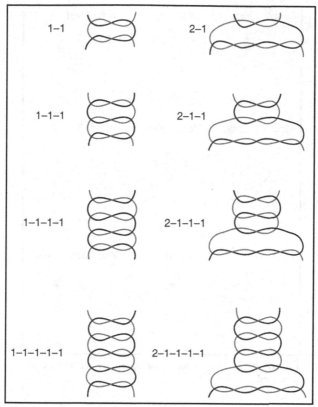

Figure 20-1. The eight parallel knots that were tested, and the international knot nomenclature.

Results

▶ Suture material

  ▷ Nonabsorbable braided polyester and absorbable polyglactin and polyglycolic acid sutures best combined ultimate tensile strength and stiffness

  ▷ Polyglyconate and polydioxanone sutures failed only at high loads, but elongated considerably under moderate loads.

  ▷ For the same suture material:

    ≫ Increasing from size 0 to size 1 increased ultimate tensile strength by an average of 35% ± 10%

    ≫ Increasing from size 1 to size 2 increased ultimate tensile strength by an average of 30% ± 7%

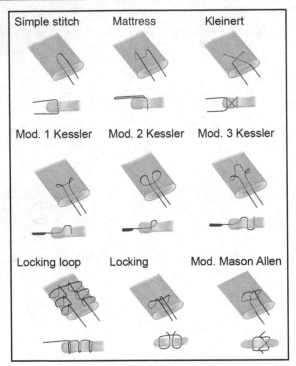

Figure 20-2. The tendon grasping suture techniques that were used.

- Knot technique
  - The 2 = 1 and the 1 = 1 knots both slipped badly, but the 1 = 1 = 1 knots of Ethibond 3 and Tevdek II 1 only slipped under loads close to the ultimate tensile strength.
  - Ethibond 3 and 1 and Tevdek II 1 were both locked securely by either the 1 = 1 = 1 = 1 or the 2 = 1 = 1 knot configurations.
  - More knots did not significantly change either elongation or ultimate tensile strength.
- Tendon-grasping technique
  - Tendon grasping with a simple stitch technique was mechanically poor.
    - Repairs with 2 simple stitches failed at 184 N.
    - Repairs with 4 simple stitches failed at 208 N.
  - A new modification of the Mason-Allen suture technique improved the ultimate tensile strength to 359 N for 2 stitches.
  - The other techniques showed intermediate results with a tendency to slip, especially in thinner tendons.

▷ Simple stitch, mattress stitch, and augmented first modification of the Kessler stitch (augmented with a 1.4-mm-thick absorbable polymembrane) were significantly less strong than the others ($P < 0.05$).

▶ Bone anchorage technique

▷ The 4-hole metal plate with a cortical graft was unsatisfactory, with the tendon slipping out at 140 ± 31 N.

▷ The metallic brush grasped the tendon better (299 ± 59 N), but the tendons were cut longitudinally and slipped out under higher loads.

▷ The Mitek G II anchor pulled out of osteoporotic bone at 142 ± 55 N.

▷ Single transosseous sutures, double transosseous sutures, and suture anchor fixation all failed at low tensile loads (about 140 N).

▷ Using a 2-mm-thick, platelike polymembrane augmentation device improved the failure strength to 329 N.

Conclusions

▶ The mechanical properties of many current repair techniques are poor.

▶ They can be greatly improved by using good materials, an improved tendon-grasping suture, and augmentation at the bone attachment.

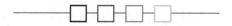

FEATURED ARTICLE

Authors: Harryman DT, Mack LA, Wang KY, Jackins SE, Richardson ML, Matsen FA 3rd.

Title: Repairs of the rotator cuff: correlation of functional results with integrity of the cuff.

Journal Information: *J Bone Joint Surg Am.* 1991;73:982–989.

A Top 100 Cited Articles in Clinical Orthopedic Sports Medicine

---

Study Design: Retrospective Review

▶ Purpose: To correlate the functional outcome of rotator cuff repairs with the integrity of the repaired cuff follow-up

▶ 105 operative repairs of rotator cuff tears in 89 patients

▸ Authors noted that 2 prior studies that attempted to make such a correlation involved few patients and led to conflicting conclusions
▸ Average follow-up 5 years, all with minimum 2-year follow-up
▸ Average age at time of repair 60 years (32 to 80 years)
▸ 86 shoulders (82%) had no history of prior cuff repair.
▸ 19 shoulders (18%) had undergone a prior cuff repair and had a second or recurrent tear repaired.
  ▷ Average time from initial to repeat repair 2 years (5 months to 11 years)
▸ Integrity of rotator cuff determined by ultrasonography at follow-up
▸ Correlated the functional result with the cuff integrity
▸ Functional evaluation based on system of the ASES
  ▷ Patient rating of comfort and satisfaction on a scale of 0 to 5
  ▷ Ranges of active and passive motion
  ▷ Evaluation of thirteen upper extremity functions
  ▷ Isometric shoulder strength measurements

Results

▸ 80% of repairs of isolated supraspinatus tendon tears were intact at the most recent follow-up.
▸ More than 50 percent of repairs of a tear involving more than the supraspinatus tendon had a recurrent defect.
▸ Older patients and patients in whom a larger tear had been repaired had a greater frequency of recurrent defects.
▸ Most patients were more comfortable and satisfied with their result at the most recent follow-up, even when they had ultrasound evidence of a recurrent defect.
▸ Shoulder with intact repairs had better function during activities of daily living and a better active flexion compared to those that had a large recurrent defect (129 ± 20 degrees vs 71 ± 41 degrees)
▸ Similar correlations were noted for:
  ▷ Range of active external and internal rotation
  ▷ Strength of flexion, abduction, and internal rotation
▸ In shoulders with recurrent defects, the degree of functional loss was related to the size of the recurrent defect.

Conclusions

▸ The integrity of the rotator cuff at follow-up, not the tear size at time of repair, is the major determinant of outcome following operative rotator cuff tear repair.
▸ The function of the patients with an intact cuff after repair of a large tear was as good as patients with an intact cuff after repair of a small tear.

- Repair of secondary tears yields results comparable to primary tear repairs when the cuff remained intact at follow-up.
- Repair of large tears yields results comparable to repairs of small tears when the cuff remained intact at follow-up.
- The chance that repairs of large tears will remain intact is less than repairs of small tears.
- Older patients tended to have larger tears and a higher prevalence of secondary defects.
- These data suggest that the quality of the cuff tissue, its attachment to bone, and the potential for a durable repair deteriorates with age and disuse.

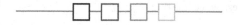

FEATURED ARTICLE

Authors: Gerber C, Fuchs B, Hodler J.

Title: The results of repair of massive tears of the rotator cuff.

Journal Information: *J Bone Joint Surg Am.* 2000;82:505–515.

A Top 100 Cited Articles in Clinical Orthopedic Sports Medicine

Study Design: Cohort Study

- Purpose:
  - ▷ To determine whether a new method of rotator cuff repair produces a lower retear rate and a better clinical outcome
  - ▷ To determine whether or not the rotator cuff muscles recover after repair
  - ▷ To correlate MRI findings with clinical results
- Prospective study of 29 patients with massive rotator cuff tears (complete detachment of at least 2 tendons)
- Cuff repaired with a new transosseous technique
  - ▷ Tendons are freed up extensively with release of the interval between the tendons to be repaired.
  - ▷ Capsulotomy performed between the capsule and the labrum from inside and the joint distracted with use of a subacromial spreader
  - ▷ Number-3 braided polyester sutures and a modified Mason-Allen tendon stitch are used.

▷ A thin titanium plate with 7 round holes is used as a cortical bone-augmentation device.

▷ Both strands of a single Mason-Allen stitch are brought through the tuberosity and through 2 holes of the plate, and the suture is tied under optimal tension over the bridge between the 2 holes of the plate.

▸ 27 patients with minimum 2-year follow-up

▸ Average follow-up 37 months (24 to 61 months)

▸ Average age 56 years (41 to 72 years), 18 men, 9 women

▸ Clinical examination

▸ Constant score

▸ Abduction strength

▸ Magnetic resonance imaging

Results

▸ Constant score (age and gender adjusted) improved from an average of 49% preop to an average of 85% post-op

▸ Post-op subjective shoulder value corresponded with 78% of that of a normal shoulder

▸ Pain-free flexion improved from an average of 92 degrees to an average of 142 degrees.

▸ Pain-free abduction improved from an average of 82 degrees to an average of 137 degrees.

▸ Significant improvement in pain ($P < 0.05$)

▸ Significant improvement in performance of activities of daily living ($P < 0.05$)

▸ The overall rate of retear was 34% (10/29).

▷ 3/9 patients who had had a posterosuperior 2-tendon tear had a retear.

▷ 2/10 patients who had had an anterosuperior 2-tendon tear had a retear.

▷ 5/10 patients who had had a 3-tendon tear had a retear.

▸ Retears occurred more often in patients with a shorter interval between the onset of the symptoms and the operation ($P < 0.05$)

▸ 17 patients with a structurally successful repair all had an excellent clinical outcome.

▸ Muscle atrophy could not be reversed except in successfully repaired supraspinatus musculotendinous units.

▸ Fatty degeneration increased in all muscles.

Conclusions

▸ The method of massive rotator cuff tear repair used in this study produced a comparatively low retear rate and good-to-excellent clinical results.

▸ The repair did not result in substantial reversal of muscular atrophy and fatty degeneration.

▶ Patients who had a retear had improvement of the shoulder compared with the preop state, but they had less improvement than did those whose repair remained structurally successful.

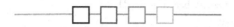

FEATURED ARTICLE

Authors: Bishop J, Kleps S, Lo IK, Bird J, Gladstone JN, Flatow EL.

Title: Cuff integrity after arthroscopic versus open rotator cuff repair: a prospective study.

Journal Information: *J Shoulder Elbow Surg.* 2006;15:290–299.

Study Design: Cohort Study

▶ Prospective study that compared post-op cuff integrity and outcome after:
  ▷ Arthroscopic rotator cuff repair (40 patients)
  ▷ Open rotator cuff repair (32 patients)
▶ Average age 64 years, 41 women, 31 men
▶ Average overall tear size:
  ▷ 2.6 cm in the open group
  ▷ 3.0 cm in the arthroscopic group
▶ Evaluations performed preoperatively and at 1 year:
  ▷ Physical examination, including dynamometer strength testing
  ▷ Magnetic resonance imaging
  ▷ SF-36
  ▷ American Shoulder and Elbow Surgeons Survey
  ▷ Constant score
  ▷ Visual analog score for pain

Results

▶ American Shoulder and Elbow Surgeons and Constant scores improved significantly in both groups ($P < 0.0001$).

- No significant overall difference in outcome measurements between the 2 groups except:
  - For tears > 3 cm, post-op external rotation strength was significantly higher in the open repair group (16.4 pounds vs 8.8 pounds, $P < 0.05$)
- 1-year cuff integrity based on MRI
  - Open group
    - 69% overall
    - 74% for tears < 3 cm
    - 62% for tears > 3cm
  - Arthroscopic group
    - 53% overall
    - 84% for tears < 3 cm
    - 24% for tears > 3 cm
- Cuff integrity for tears > 3 cm significantly higher in the open group (62% vs 24%, $P < 0.036$)
- Patients in the arthroscopic group with intact cuff compared to those who had a retear:
  - Significantly greater strength of elevation ($P < 0.01$)
  - Significantly greater strength of external rotation ($P < 0.02$)

Conclusions

- Open and arthroscopic rotator cuff repairs have similar clinical outcomes.
- For small tears (< 3 cm), cuff integrity is comparable between the 2 treatment groups.
- Large tears (> 3 cm) have twice the retear rate after arthroscopic repair.

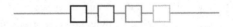

FEATURED ARTICLE

Authors: Franceschi F, Ruzzini L, Longo UG, Martina FM, Zobel BB, Maffulli N, Denaro V.

Title: Equivalent clinical results of arthroscopic single-row and double-row suture anchor repair for rotator cuff tears: a randomized controlled trial.

Journal Information: *Am J Sport Med.* 2007;35:1254–1260.

Study Design: Prospective Randomized Study

- Purpose: To compare single- and double-row arthroscopic repair techniques in patients with large and massive rotator cuff tears
  - ▷ A double row of suture anchors increases the tendon–bone contact area, reconstituting a more anatomic configuration of the rotator cuff footprint.
  - ▷ Restoring the anatomic footprint may improve the healing and mechanical strength of repaired tendons.
- 60 patients
  - ▷ 30 randomized to rotator cuff repair using a single-row suture anchor technique
    - » 4 lost to final follow-up
    - » Average age 63.5 years (43 to 76 years), 14 women, 12 men
  - ▷ 30 randomized to rotator cuff repair using a double-row suture anchor technique
    - » 4 lost to final follow-up
- Average age 59.6 years (45 to 80 years), 16 men, 10 women
- Outcome assessments
  - ▷ Modified UCLA shoulder rating scale
  - ▷ Range of motion
  - ▷ Magnetic resonance arthrography at final follow-up (2 years)
- Average follow-up 22.5 months (range 18 to 25 months)

Results

- No statistically significant difference in the UCLA shoulder score and range of motion values at 2 years
- Post-op MR arthrography at 2 years
  - ▷ No statistical difference in healing rates between 2 groups ($P > 0.05$)
  - ▷ Single-row technique
    - » 14 patients with intact tendons
    - » 10 patients with partial-thickness defects
    - » 2 patients with full-thickness defects
  - ▷ Double-row technique
    - » 18 patients with intact tendons
    - » 7 patients with partial-thickness defects
    - » 1 patient with full-thickness defect

Conclusions

- Single- and double-row techniques provide comparable clinical outcomes at 2 years.

▶ Double-row technique produces a mechanically superior construct compared with the single-row method in restoring the anatomic footprint of the rotator cuff, but these mechanical advantages do not translate into better clinical outcomes.

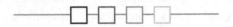

CLASSIC ARTICLE

Author: L'Episcopo JB.

Title: Tendon transplantation in obstetrical palsy.

Journal Information: *Am J Surg.* 1934;25:122–125.

Study Design: Retrospective Review

▶ Describes the L'Episcopo tendon transfer procedure used for obstetrical palsy
▶ Obstetrical palsy = brachial plexus injury (Erb palsy involving C5–C6 is the most common)
▶ Loss of muscle balance between the external and internal rotators results in an internal rotation shoulder deformity and adduction contracture.
▶ Deformity is disabling, impacting many activities of daily living
▶ Prior operations have only released contractures
▶ L'Episcipo postulated that if you could permanently strengthen the external rotators and weaken the internal rotators, you could prevent deformity recurrence and improve function.
▶ L'Episcipo tendon transfer is always done in conjunction with the Sever procedure
▶ Sever procedure = release of the subscapularis and pectoralis major muscles to address the shoulder adduction contracture
▶ L'Episcipo procedure = teres major tendon is detached and transferred to a location more lateral on the proximal humeral shaft
▶ New insertion site is almost directly opposite its original insertion, producing shoulder external rotation when the muscle contracts.
▶ After surgery, plaster of Paris spica cast applied with the arm abducted, externally rotated, and the forearm flexed and supinated

Results

▶ Reported on 6 patients treated with this transfer, all of whom showed marked functional improvement

▶ Noted that patients with longest follow-up showed the most improvement, suggesting that the transferred muscle strength gradually improves

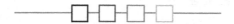

FEATURED ARTICLE

Authors: Mansat P, Cofield RH, Kerstien TE, Rowland CM.

Title: Complications of rotator cuff repair.

Journal Information: *Orthop Clin of North Am.* 1997;28:205–213.

Study Design: Retrospective Review

▶ 116 shoulders undergoing rotator cuff repair

▶ Average age 57 years (21 to 84 years), 80 men, 36 women

▶ Average follow-up 23 months (1 to 108 months)

▶ Complications categorized as medical or surgical

  ▷ All medical complications occurred during the hospitalization period.

  ▷ Surgical complications within 6 weeks of surgery were defined as early.

  ▷ Surgical complications > 6 weeks after surgery were defined as late.

  ▷ Surgical complications that did not affect the final result or that did not require significant additional treatment were categorized as minor.

  ▷ Surgical complications that affected the final result or required significant additional treatment were categorized as major.

Results

▶ 38% (44 patients) developed complications.

▶ 12% (14 patients) developed a medical complication.

  ▷ 5 urinary complications (urinary tract infection, urinary retention, urethral bleeding)

  ▷ 3 pulmonary complications (pneumonia, tracheopharyngitis)

  ▷ 2 gastrointestinal complications (gastric hemorrhage due to gastric ulcers)

  ▷ 2 metabolic complications (hyponatremia, acute gouty attack)

> ▷ 1 cardiac complication (cardiac arrhythmia)
> ▷ 1 pulmonary embolism
> ▶ 33% (38 patients) developed a surgical complication.
> ▶ 8 patients had more than one surgical complication.
> ▶ 23 major surgical complications developed that affected the final result
>   ▷ 17 failure of rotator cuff tendon repair
>   ▷ 3 frozen shoulders
>   ▷ 2 deep infections
>   ▷ 1 dislocation
> ▶ Risk factors associated with the development of a complication were:
>   ▷ Age
>   ▷ Prior surgery
>   ▷ A lesser degree of preop active elevation, passive elevation, or external rotation
>   ▷ More pronounced preop weakness in abduction, flexion, or internal rotation
>   ▷ Narrowed acromiohumeral interval (strong association between acromiohumeral interval < 7 mm and development of a post-op complication)
>   ▷ Absence of a distal clavicle excision
>   ▷ Larger tear size

Conclusions

> ▶ It can be anticipated that failure of tendon repair healing will occur in a variable number of patients following surgery.
> ▶ The frequency of complications seems to parallel the frequency following other major musculoskeletal operative procedures.
> ▶ To reduce complications, the surgeon should focus on enhancing the consistency of tendon healing following rotator cuff repair.

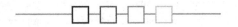

FEATURED ARTICLE

Authors: Neviaser RJ, Neviaser TJ.

Title: Reoperation for failed rotator cuff repair: analysis of fifty cases.

Journal Information: *J Shoulder Elbow Surg.* 1992;1:283–286.

Study Design: Retrospective Review

- ▶ Purpose: To analyze cases of reoperation for failed cuff repair to determine whether or not functional improvement can be achieved
- ▶ 50 patients who underwent reoperation for failure of previous repair of rotator cuff tear
- ▶ Average age at the time of the final reoperation 54.5 years (34 to 79 years)
- ▶ Average number of prior operations 1.6 (1 to 4)
  - ▷ 30 patients had undergone one prior operation.
  - ▷ 13 patients had undergone 2 prior operations.
  - ▷ 4 patients had undergone 3 prior operations.
  - ▷ 3 patients had undergone 4 prior operations.
- ▶ Average follow-up after final repair 30 months (24 to 84 months)
- ▶ Evaluated pain, motion, strength, and patient satisfaction

Results

- ▶ Pain
  - ▷ 92% (46 patients) reported pain improvement.
  - ▷ 8% (4 patients) were unchanged.
- ▶ Motion
  - ▷ 52% (26 patients) showed an average increase in elevation of 50 degrees (10 to 130 degrees)
  - ▷ 44% (22 patients) showed no improvement from their preop motion.
  - ▷ 4% (2 patients) lost an average of 45 degrees of their preop motion, but still had more than 90 degrees.
  - ▷ Overall mean elevation increased from 92 to 137 degrees.
  - ▷ 17% had < 90 degrees of motion before surgery.
  - ▷ Only 6 patients had < 90 degrees of motion after surgery, and all had deltoid abnormalities.
- ▶ Strength
  - ▷ Only 26/50 had preop strength assessment
  - ▷ Average preop strength in external rotation 3+ (3 to 4)
  - ▷ Average post-op strength in external rotation 4+ (4 to 5–)
  - ▷ Average preop strength in elevation 3+ (3 to 4)
  - ▷ Average post-op strength in elevation 4+ (4 to 5–)
- ▶ Satisfaction
  - ▷ 90% (45 patients) were satisfied with their results.
  - ▷ 10% (5 patients) were dissatisfied.
- ▶ Rupture size, number of prior operations, and biceps dysfunction did not affect the result.

- ▶ Factors associated with success:
  - ▷ Adequate decompression
  - ▷ Closure of all defects with tendon-to-bone junctures (by direct repair, interpositional grafting, or local tendon transfers)
  - ▷ Avoiding use of weights or resistive exercises during the early (first 3 months) post-op rehabilitation period
  - ▷ Intact, functioning deltoid

Conclusions

- ▶ Reoperation for failed cuff repair can result in decreased pain and increased motion.
- ▶ Important factors in achieving success include adequate decompression and careful mobilization and closure of the rotator cuff to bone.
- ▶ Proper post-op rehabilitation with early passive mobility at 48 hours after surgery and avoidance of the use of weights in the early phase also contributes to success.

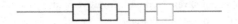

FEATURED ARTICLE

Author: Wiley M.

Title: Superior humeral dislocation. A complication following decompression and debridement for rotator cuff tears.

Journal Information: *Clin Orthop.* 1991;263:135–141.

Study Design: Retrospective Review

- ▶ Author describes 4 cases in which there was superior humeral head migration following failed rotator cuff repairs
- ▶ This complication can also occur following debridement and release of the subacromial bursa in irreparable rotator cuff tears.

Results

- ▶ Reported on 2 cases where efforts were taken to reestablish the roof of the bursa

- Screwed a 7.5-cm rectangle of harvested iliac crest to the coracoid and to the undersurface of the acromion to reestablish the subacromial arch
- 76-year-old female who was status post revision total shoulder arthroplasty and failed rotator cuff repair whose humeral head protruded forward and upward beneath the skin
  ▷ Patient pleased and free of pain, although abduction and forward flexion impossible
  ▷ Patient list to long-term follow-up
- 64-year-old woman also status post revision shoulder arthroplasty with an irreparable rotator cuff whose humeral head subluxed superiorly
  ▷ Short-term (< 1 year) follow-up
  ▷ Significant pain relief
  ▷ 40 degrees of forward flexion and 40 degrees of abduction

Conclusions

- Debridement alone should rarely be performed for massive rotator cuff tears, as it may lead to upward dislocation of the humeral head and increased disability.
- For late repair of superior dislocations, the author recommends repairing the rotator cuff by transposition, slide, or graft and reestablishing the roof of the bursa with a bone graft.

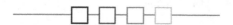

FEATURED ARTICLE

Authors: Mohtadi NG, Hollinshead RM, Sasyniuk TM, Fletcher JA, Chan DS, Li FX.

Title: A randomized clinical trial comparing open to arthroscopic acromioplasty with mini-open rotator cuff repair for full-thickness rotator cuff tears: disease-specific quality of life outcome at an average 2-year follow-up.

Journal Information: *Am J Sports Med.* 2008;36:1043–1051.

2006 AAOSM O'Donoghue Award Winner

Study Design: Prospective Randomized Study

- Purpose: To compare 2 surgical procedures—standard open acromioplasty with rotator cuff repair (open) vs arthroscopic acromioplasty with mini-open rotator cuff repair (scope mini-open)
  - ▷ Deltoid dehiscence is a potential complication of open acromioplasty and rotator cuff repair.
  - ▷ The advantage of combining arthroscopic acromioplasty with a mini-open repair is the preservation of the deltoid origin.
- Patients with full-thickness rotator cuff tears who had unremitting pain and who had failed nonoperative treatment randomized to:
  - ▷ Open repair (29 patients analyzed)
  - ▷ Scope mini-open repair (30 patients analyzed)
- Excluded massive irreparable cuff tears
- Study performed at 5 centers with a total of 6 surgeons

Assessments

- Performed at baseline, 3 and 6 months, and 1 and 2 years
- Disease-specific rotator cuff quality of life index (maximum score of 100 representing a high quality of life)
- American Shoulder and Elbow Society score
- Shoulder rating questionnaire
- Functional shoulder elevation test

Results

- Mean rotator cuff quality of life scores at an average follow-up of 28 months were not statistically different.
  - ▷ Open, 86.9 (95% confidence interval: 81.8 to 92.0)
  - ▷ Scope mini-open, 87.2 (95% confidence interval: 80.6 to 93.8)
- At 3 months, the patients who underwent scope mini-open showed statistically significant better outcomes (55.6 vs 71.3; $P = 0.005$).
- The baseline to 3-month difference in rotator cuff quality of life scores between the scope mini-open and open groups was also statistically significant.

Results

- Patient outcomes improved from baseline to all post-op measurement intervals.
- The quality of life of patients undergoing the arthroscopic acromioplasty with mini-open rotator cuff repair improved statistically significantly and clinically at 3 months compared with the open group.

► No difference in outcome at 1 and 2 years after surgery between the scope mini-open and open procedures

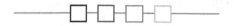

FEATURED ARTICLE

Authors: Miller BS, Downie BK, Kohen RB, Kijek T, Lesniak B, Jacobson JA, Hughes RE, Carpenter JE.

Title: When do rotator cuff repairs fail? Serial ultrasound examination after arthroscopic repair of large and massive rotator cuff tears.

Journal Information: *Am J Sports Med.* 2011;39:2064–2070.

2010 AAOSM O'Donoghue Award Winner

Study Design: Cohort Study

► 22 consecutive patients with large (> 3 cm) rotator cuff tears who underwent arthroscopic repair
► Average age 63.7 years, 11 men, 11 women
► Surgical indication was either:
  ▷ Failure of a 3-month course of nonoperative management (home or clinic-based therapy program)
  ▷ A known traumatic rotator cuff rupture in a previously asymptomatic shoulder
► Serial ultrasound examinations performed at 2 days, 2 weeks, 6 weeks, 3 months, 6 months, 12 months, and 24 months after surgery
► Patient self-assessment at 6, 12, and 24 months
  ▷ Western Ontario Rotator Cuff (WORC) Index scores

Results

► 41% (9/22) of repairs demonstrated a recurrent rotator cuff tear.
  ▷ 7 retears occurred within 3 months of surgery.
  ▷ 2 retears occurred between 3 and 6 months after surgery.

- At 24-month follow-up, WORC scores favoring intact rotator cuffs over retears approached statistical significance ($P = 0.07$).
  - ▷ Mean WORC for patients with intact rotator cuff 123.9
  - ▷ Mean WORC for patients with retear 659.8

Conclusions

- Recurrent tears are not uncommon after arthroscopic repair of large and massive rotator cuff tears.
- Recurrent tears appear to occur more frequently in the early post-op period (within the first 3 months) and are associated with inferior clinical outcomes.

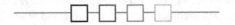

REVIEW ARTICLES

Burkhart SS. Current concepts: reconciling the paradox of rotator cuff tear versus debridement: a unified biomechanical rationale for the treatment of rotator cuff tears. *Arthroscopy*. 1994;10:4–19.

Burkhart SS, Lo IKY. Arthroscopic rotator cuff repair. *J Am Acad Orthop Surg*. 2006;14:333–346.

Gerber C, Hersche O. Tendon transfers for the treatment of irreparable rotator cuff defects. *Orthop Clin North Am*. 1997;28:195–203.

Wolff, AB, Sethi, P, Sutton KM, Covey AS, Magit DP, Medvecky M. Partial-thickness rotator cuff tears. *J Am Acad Orthop Surg*. 2006;14:715–725.

Proximal Biceps Tendon Injuries

Chapter *21*

FEATURED ARTICLE

Authors: Snyder SJ, Karzel RP, Del Pizzo W, Ferkel RD, Friedman MJ.

Title: SLAP lesions of the shoulder.

Journal Information: *Arthroscopy.* 1990;6:274–279.

Study Design: Retrospective Review

▸ More than 700 shoulder arthroscopies
▸ Identified a specific pattern of injury to the superior labrum of the shoulder in 27 patients
▸ Labeled this injury pattern a "SLAP lesion"
  ▷ SLAP = superior labrum anterior and posterior
▸ Superior labral injury begins posteriorly and spreads anteriorly, stopping before or at the midglenoid notch, and includes the "anchor" of the biceps tendon to the labrum
▸ Average age of these 27 patients 37.5 years (20 to 60 years), 23 men, 4 women
▸ Mechanism of injury
  ▷ Most common: Compression force to the shoulder, usually due to a fall onto an outstretched arm, with the shoulder in abduction and slight forward flexion at impact
  ▷ Traction on the arm, either due to a sudden pull on the arm or as a result of throwing or of an overhead sports motion

Miller MD, Mauffrey C, Hak DJ.
Rapid Reference Review in Sports Medicine:
Pivotal Papers Revealed (pp 249-253).
© 2016 Taylor & Francis Group.

- ▸ Clinical complaints
  - ▹ Pain, greater with overhead activity
  - ▹ Painful shoulder "catching" or "popping"
- ▸ No preop imaging test accurately defined the superior labral pathology.

Results

- ▸ Superior labrum anterior and posterior lesions can only be diagnosed arthroscopically.
- ▸ Divided pathology into 4 distinct types
  - ▹ Type I—3 patients (11%)
    - » Marked fraying of the superior labrum with a degenerative appearance
    - » Peripheral labral edge remained firmly attached to the glenoid
    - » Intact attachment of the biceps tendon to the labrum
  - ▹ Type II—11 patients (41%)
    - » Fraying and degenerative changes (like type I)
    - » Superior labrum and attached biceps tendon were also stripped off the glenoid, making the labral-biceps anchor unstable and arched away from the glenoid.
  - ▹ Type III—9 patients (33%)
    - » Superior labral bucket-handle tear
    - » Central portion of the tear was displaceable into the joint
    - » Peripheral portion of the labrum firmly attached to the glenoid and to the biceps tendon
    - » Biceps tendon intact
  - ▹ Type IV—4 patients (15%)
    - » Bucket-handle superior labral tear (like in type III)
    - » Tear also extended into the biceps tendon
    - » Attached partial tear of the biceps tendon tended to displace with the labral flap into the joint
- ▸ High incidence of associated pathology
  - ▹ 26% (7 patients) had a partial-thickness rotator cuff tear.
  - ▹ 15% (4 patients) had a full-thickness rotator cuff tear.
  - ▹ 15% (4 patients) had anterior instability.
  - ▹ 15% (4 patients) had humeral head chondromalacia or an indentation fracture.
  - ▹ 11% (3 patients) had acromioclavicular joint arthritis.
- ▸ Treatment
  - ▹ Superior labrum anterior and posterior lesion treated arthroscopically in all patients

▷ 12 patients (48%) had primarily a SLAP lesion and were treated arthroscopically.

▷ 3 patients (11%) had primarily a SLAP lesion but also underwent an arthroscopically assisted open biceps tenodesis.

▷ 9 patients (33%) also had open procedures for repair of major associated pathology.

▷ 2 patients (7%) had additional arthroscopic procedures for repair of major associated pathology.

▶ 1 complication with an ultimate fair result

▷ Arthroscopically placed staple felt to show impingement into the joint on x-ray, so patient returned to operating room for open staple removal and biceps tenodesis—subsequently developed arthrofibrosis requiring manipulation

Conclusions

▶ The SLAP lesion causes significant disability.

▶ The SLAP lesion is only diagnosable by arthroscopic examination.

▶ Pathology was successfully treated (preliminary findings based on short-term follow-up) in a high percentage of cases by arthroscopic techniques.

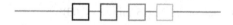

FEATURED ARTICLE

Authors: McMahon PJ, Burkhart A, Musahl V, Debski RE.

Title: Glenohumeral translations are increased after a type II superior labrum anterior-posterior lesion: a cadaveric study of severity of passive stabilizer injury.

Journal Information: *J Shoulder Elbow Surg.* 2004;13:39–44.

Study Design: Cadaveric Study

▶ Purpose: To determine whether the severity of type II SLAP lesions affected glenohumeral joint translations

▶ 8 cadaveric specimens studied

- Examined 2 type II slap lesions of different severity
  - ▷ Superior labrum and the biceps anchor elevated subperiosteally off the glenoid (SLAP-II-1)
  - ▷ Biceps anchor completely detached (SLAP-II-2)
- Simulated anterior and posterior load and shift tests applied using a robotic/ universal force-moment sensor testing system
- Simulated apprehension test for anterior instability performed by applying a 50 N anterior load with a 3 Nm external rotation torque at 30 and 60 degrees of abduction
- Loading was first performed on an intact shoulder that was vented to atmospheric pressure and then repeated after creating one of two type II SLAP lesions.

Results

Anterior Loading

- Anterior translation with anterior load at 30 degrees abduction
  - ▷ Significantly increased anterior translation between vented joint and SLAP lesions ($P = 0.03$)
  - ▷ Vented joint: 18.5 ± 8.5 mm
  - ▷ SLAP-II-1 lesion: 25.0 ± 6.8 mm ($P = 0.03$)
  - ▷ SLAP-II-2 lesion: 26.2 ± 6.5 mm ($P = 0.03$)
- Anterior translation with anterior load at 60 degrees abduction
  - ▷ No significant difference between vented joint and SLAP lesions
  - ▷ Vented joint: 16.6 ± 9.6 mm
  - ▷ SLAP-II-1 lesion: 18.8 ± 9.6 mm
  - ▷ SLAP-II-2 lesion: 19.4 ± 10.1 mm
- Inferior translation was also seen with anterior loading.
- Inferior translation with anterior load at 30 degrees of abduction
  - ▷ Significantly increased inferior translation between vented joint and SLAP-II-2 lesions ($P = 0.05$)
  - ▷ Vented joint: 3.8 ± 4.0 mm
  - ▷ SLAP-II-1 lesion: 7.8 ± 4.9 mm
  - ▷ SLAP-II-2 lesion: 8.5 ± 5.4 mm ($P = 0.05$)

Posterior Loading

- Posterior translation with posterior load at 30 degrees of abduction
  - ▷ Significantly increased posterior translation between vented joint and SLAP lesions
  - ▷ Vented joint: 15.3 ± 8.4 mm

▷ SLAP-II-1 lesion: 15.9 ± 8.4 mm ($P = 0.037$)

▷ SLAP-II-2 lesion: 16.2 ± 8.3 mm ($P = 0.029$)

▶ Posterior translation with posterior load at 60 degrees of abduction

▷ No significant difference between vented joint and SLAP lesions

▷ Vented joint: 11.1 ± 8.4 mm

▷ SLAP-II-1 lesion: 11.3 ± 8.0 mm ($P = 0.037$)

▷ SLAP-II-2 lesion: 12.2 ± 8.0 mm ($P = 0.029$)

Combined Loading

▶ No significant increase in anterior translation with combined anterior and external rotation loading between the 2 SLAP lesions

Conclusions

▶ Glenohumeral translations increased in simulated type II SLAP lesions, regardless of the lesion severity.

▶ Passive stabilizers that are injured in type II SLAP lesions, as well as dynamic activity in the long head of the biceps tendon, should be considered during stabilizing surgical procedures.

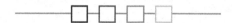

REVIEW ARTICLE

Barber FA, Field LD, Ryu RKN. Instructional course lectures: biceps tendon and superior labral injuries: decision making. *J Bone Joint Surg Am.* 1007;89:1844–1855.

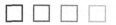

Acromioclavicular Disorders

Chapter **22**

FEATURED ARTICLE

Authors: Fukuda K, Craug EV, An KN, Cofield RH, Chao EY.

Title: Biomechanical study of the ligamentous system of the acromioclavicular joint.

Journal Information: *J Bone Joint Surg.* 1986;68:434–440.

Study Design: Cadaveric Study

▸ Purpose: To determine the contribution of the acromioclavicular and coracoclavicular ligaments to acromioclavicular joint stability

▸ Twelve cadaveric specimens studied

  ▷ Gross examination of ligaments

  ▷ Changes in ligament length under applied load

  ▷ Twelve modes of joint displacement were examined.

  ▷ Sequential ligament sectioning and load-displacement testing

▸ Anatomic structures supporting the acromioclavicular joint

  ▷ Acromioclavicular ligament

  ▷ Coracoclavicular ligament

    » Conoid ligament

    » Trapezoid ligament

▸ Distances between insertions at various extreme positions of the clavicle were studied with biplane radiographs.

Miller MD, Mauffrey C, Hak DJ.
Rapid Reference Review in Sports Medicine:
Pivotal Papers Revealed (pp 255-259).
© 2016 Taylor & Francis Group.

Results

▸ Acromioclavicular ligament is the primary constraint for posterior displacement of the clavicle and posterior axial rotation

▸ Conoid ligament appeared more important than previously described

▸ Conoid ligament is primary constraint for anterior and superior rotation, as well as anterior and superior clavicle displacement

▸ Trapezoid ligament contributed less constraint to clavicle movement in both horizontal and vertical planes, except when the clavicle moved in axial compression toward the acromion process

▸ Contributions of different ligaments to constraint changed with the direction of joint displacement and with the amount of loading and displacement

▸ For many directions of displacement:

  ▷ Acromioclavicular joint contributed a greater amount to constraint at smaller degrees of displacement

  ▷ Coracoclavicular ligaments (primarily the conoid ligament) contributed a greater amount of constraint with larger amounts of displacement

Conclusions/Clinical Relevance

▸ All of the ligaments supporting the acromioclavicular joint provide a substantial contribution to joint stability.

▸ Contribution to stability changes with the direction and amount of loading

▸ To allow maximum healing strength following an acromioclavicular joint injury, all ligaments should be allowed to participate in the healing process.

▸ Some repair methods, such as those that include distal clavicle excision, may not make this possible.

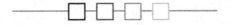

FEATURED ARTICLE

Authors: Schlegel TF, Burks RT, Marcus R, Dunn HK.

Title: A prospective evaluation of untreated grade III AC separations.

Journal Information: *Am J Sports Med.* 2001;29:699–703.

Study Design: Cohort Study

- Purpose: To document the natural history of nonoperatively treated acute grade III acromioclavicular separation
- Prospective study of 25 patients with an acute grade III acromioclavicular separation treated nonoperatively
- Sling for comfort and progressive early range of motion
- No formal physical therapy
- Examined at 6, 12, 24, 36, and 52 weeks
- Outcome assessments
  - ▷ Subjective questionnaire
    - ≫ Visual analog scale
      - ⟩ Degree of pain
      - ⟩ Functional disability
      - ⟩ Stiffness
      - ⟩ Strength
      - ⟩ Cosmetic appearance
      - ⟩ Overall satisfaction
  - ▷ Isometric dynamometer strength testing
  - ▷ Military press and bench press strength testing
- Also performed strength testing on 10 uninjured subjects to evaluate dominant-to-nondominant side strength differences
- Follow-up
  - ▷ 20/25 patients completed the 1-year evaluation
  - ▷ 1 patient underwent surgical repair at 2 weeks because of cosmetic concerns.
  - ▷ 4 patients did not complete the 1-year strength evaluation, but were contacted by phone and all 4 had returned to work, denied any functional limitations, and were satisfied with their outcome.

Results

- Average length of sling use 8 days (2 to 25 days)
- Analgesic medications required for < 1 week in 15 patients and no more than 2 weeks in the remaining 5 patients
- Average time until return to work 9 days (1 to 24 days)
- Subjective outcome
  - ▷ 80% (16/20) rated overall subjective results favorable
  - ▷ 20% (4/20) rated their outcome suboptimal
    - ≫ For 3 of these patients, their dissatisfaction was not enough to warrant surgery.
- No limitation of shoulder motion

- Strength testing
  - ▷ No difference between sides in rotational shoulder muscle strength
  - ▷ Only the bench press showed a significant side-to-side difference ($P < 0.05$).
    - » Average 17% weaker on the injured side
- Residual deformity was unacceptable in 20% (5/25) of the original group.
  - ▷ 1 patient underwent surgery at 2 weeks.
  - ▷ 1 patient underwent Weaver-Dunn procedure at 18 months.
  - ▷ The other 3 did not pursue further operative treatment.

Conclusions

- The majority of patients with type III acromioclavicular separations will do well without any formal treatment.
- A small percentage of patients will require delayed surgical intervention, but it is unclear from this study which patients may have a poor outcome from nonoperative treatment.
- This study provides a reference with which to judge proposed operative treatment of acute grade III acromioclavicular separations.

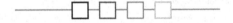

CLASSIC ARTICLE
Authors: Weaver JK, Dunn HK.
Title: Treatment of acromioclavicular injuries, especially complete acromioclavicular separation.
Journal Information: *J Bone Joint Surg Am.* 1972;54:1187–1194.

Study Design: Retrospective Review

- Original description of distal clavicle excision and transfer of coracoacromial ligament into the medullary canal (now known as the Weaver-Dunn procedure)
- Report on 12 acute and 3 chronic injuries
- Average follow-up 35 months (16 to 52 months)

▶ Outcome evaluation

  ▷ Good = full range of motion, no pain, good cosmetic result

  ▷ Fair = slight fatigue pain, residual deformity, slight loss of full elevation of the arm

  ▷ Poor = significant pain, loss of motion, gross deformity or need for second operative procedure

Results

▶ Outcome

  ▷ 11 good

  ▷ 3 fair

    » These cases, which were early in the series before adequate shortening of the coracoacromial ligament was emphasized, had incomplete reduction of the clavicular deformity but had no pain, weakness, or loss of motion.

  ▷ 1 poor

    » Patient had sudden pain and recurrence of deformity 16 months post op

▶ Patients with acute and chronic type III acromioclavicular separations should be treated with this new operation that combines distal clavicle resection and suture of the coracoacromial ligament into the intramedullary canal to achieve anatomic clavicle reduction.

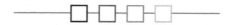

REVIEW ARTICLE

Simovitch R, Sanders B, Ozbaydar M, Lavery K, Warner JJ. Acromioclavicular joint injuries: diagnosis and management. *J Am Acad Orthop Surg.* 2009;17:207–219.

Adhesive Capsulitis

Chapter 23

FEATURED ARTICLE

Authors: Dodenhoff RM, Levy O, Wilson A, Copeland SA.

Title: Manipulation under anesthesia for primary frozen shoulder: effect on early recovery and return to activity.

Journal Information: *J Shoulder Elbow Surg.* 2000;9:23–26.

Study Design: Cohort Study

▶ Prospective study of assessed 39 shoulders in 37 patients with a diagnosis of primary frozen shoulder
  ▷ Traditionally, frozen shoulder regarded as a self-limiting condition, lasting 18 to 30 months
▶ Purpose:
  ▷ To assess the effectiveness of manipulation under anesthesia in the management of primary frozen shoulder in restoring function as measured with the Constant score
  ▷ To assess the effect of manipulation on restoration of range of motion
  ▷ To assess patient satisfaction with the procedure
▶ Mean age 53 years (33 to 63 years), 27 women, 10 men
▶ Treated with manipulation under anesthesia
▶ Mean telephone follow-up 11 months (6 to 18 months)

Miller MD, Mauffrey C, Hak DJ.
Rapid Reference Review in Sports Medicine:
Pivotal Papers Revealed (pp 261-267).
© 2016 Taylor & Francis Group.

Results

- No complications were seen.
- Median Constant score
  - Preop 24
  - 3 to 6 weeks postmanipulation 63
  - 3 months postmanipulation 69
  - Improvement was maintained at final telephone follow-up.
- Range of motion
  - Abduction
    - » Preop 60 degrees
    - » 3 to 6 weeks postmanipulation 120 degrees
  - External rotation
    - » Preop 20 degrees
    - » 3 to 6 weeks postmanipulation 50 degrees
- At 3 months
  - 59% (23 shoulders) no or mild disability
  - 28.2% (11 shoulders) moderate degree of disability
  - 2.8% (5 shoulders) severe degree of disability
- Overall, 94% of patients were satisfied with the procedure.
- No relationship between the initial Constant score or the initial range of motion after manipulation and the final result

Conclusions

- Manipulation under anesthesia results in significant improvement in early shoulder function in patients with primary frozen shoulder.
- It is a simple, well-tolerated procedure with high patient satisfaction and low complications.
- The authors recommend its use in reducing the duration of morbidity seen in this distressing, confusing, and frustrating condition.

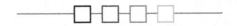

FEATURED ARTICLE

Authors: Jacobs LG, Smith MG, Khan SA, Smith K, Joshi M.

Title: Manipulation or intra-articular steroids in the management of adhesive capsulitis of the shoulder? A prospective randomized trial.

Journal Information: *J Shoulder Elbow Surg.* 2009;18:348–353.

Study Design: Prospective Randomized Study

- ▶ 53 patients with idiopathic "primary" frozen shoulder randomized to:
  - ▷ Manipulation under anesthesia (28 patients)
  - ▷ Series of 3 steroid injections and 5 cc air distention at 6-week intervals (25 patients)
- ▶ Average age 56.7 years, 35 women, 18 men
- ▶ Follow-up at 2, 6, and 12 weeks and at 6, 9, 12, 18, and 24 months
- ▶ Outcome measurements
  - ▷ Constant score
  - ▷ Visual analogue score
  - ▷ SF-36

Result

- ▶ No statistical differences in outcome measurements between the 2 treatment groups

Conclusions

- ▶ The authors recommend treatment using steroid injections with distension as an outpatient for the treatment of idiopathic "primary" frozen shoulder.
- ▶ Steroid injections with distension have the same clinical outcome as a manipulation under anesthesia with fewer risks.

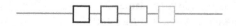

FEATURED ARTICLE

Authors: Quraishi NA, Johnston P, Bayer J, Crowe M, Chakrabarti AJ.

Title: Thawing the frozen shoulder. A randomised trial comparing manipulation under anaesthesia with hydrodilatation.

Journal Information: *J Bone Joint Surg Br.* 2007;89:1197–1200.

Study Design: Prospective Randomized Study

- 36 patients (38 shoulders) with adhesive capsulitis in stage II of the disease process randomized to:
  - Manipulation under anesthesia (18 shoulders, 17 patients)
  - Hydrodilatation (20 shoulders, 19 patients)
- Hydrodilatation performed by radiologist under fluoroscopy with injection of 10 to 55 mL or radiopaque contrast material until the capsule ruptured
- Mean age 55.2 years (44 to 70 years), 21 women, 15 men
- Mean symptom duration 33.7 weeks (12 to 76 weeks)
- Outcome measurements
  - Visual analog score for pain
  - Constant score
  - Range of motion
  - Patient satisfaction

Results

- Visual analog score
  - Manipulation under anesthesia treatment group
    - 5.7 (3 to 8.5) prior to treatment
    - 4.7 (0 to 8.5) at 2 months ($P = 0.02$)
    - 2.7 (0 to 9) at 6 months ($P = 0.0006$)
  - Hydrodilatation treatment group
    - 6.1 (4 to 10) prior to treatment
    - 2.4 (0 to 8) at 2 months ($P = 0.001$)
    - 1.7 (0 to 7) at 6 months ($P = 0.0006$)
  - Visual analog scores in hydrodilatation treatment group significantly better than manipulation under anesthesia group over the 6-month follow-up period ($P < 0.0001$)

▶ Mean Constant score
   ▷ Manipulation under anesthesia treatment group
     » 36 (26 to 66) prior to treatment
     » 58.5 (24 to 90) at 2 months ($P = 0.001$)
     » 59.5 (23 to 85) at 6 months ($P = 0.0006$)
   ▷ Hydrodilatation treatment group
     » 28.8 (18 to 55) prior to treatment
     » 57.4 (17 to 80) at 2 months ($P = 0.0004$)
     » 65.9 (28 to 92) at 6 months ($P = 0.0005$)
   ▷ Constant scores in hydrodilatation treatment group significantly better than manipulation under anesthesia group over the 6-month follow-up period ($P = 0.02$)
▶ Range of motion improved in all patients over the 6 months, but no significant difference between the 2 groups
▶ Satisfaction at final follow-up
   ▷ 94% (17/18 patients) in hydrodilatation group satisfied or very satisfied
   ▷ 81% (13/16 patients) in manipulation group satisfied or very satisfied

Conclusion

▶ Although most patients were treated successfully by either method, patients treated by hydrodilatation did better than those treated by manipulation under anesthesia.

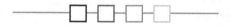

FEATURED ARTICLE

Authors: Russell S, Jariwala A, Conlon R, Selfe J, Richards J, Walton M.

Title: A blinded, randomized, controlled trial assessing conservative management strategies for frozen shoulder.

Journal Information: *J Shoulder Elbow Surg.* 2014;23:500–507.

Study Design: Prospective Randomized Study

- ▶ 75 patients with idiopathic frozen shoulder randomly assigned to 1 of 3 groups
  - ▷ Group exercise class
  - ▷ Individual physiotherapy
  - ▷ Home exercises alone
- ▶ Mean age 51.1 years (40 to 65 years), 35 women, 40 men
- ▶ Mean symptom duration 5.79 months (4 to 10 months)
- ▶ Outcome measurements at baseline, 6 weeks, 6 months, and 1 year
  - ▷ Made by a single independent physiotherapist who was blinded to the treatment groups
  - ▷ Range of motion
  - ▷ Constant score
  - ▷ Oxford Shoulder Score
  - ▷ SF-36
  - ▷ Hospital Anxiety and Disability Scale (HADS) outcome measures

Results

- ▶ Significant improvement in both Constant and Oxford scores for all treatment groups between the different time intervals ($P < 0.001$)
- ▶ Mean Constant score
  - ▷ Exercise class group
    - ≫ 39.8 at baseline
    - ≫ 71.5 (60 to 89) at 6 weeks
    - ≫ 88.1 (71 to 96) at 1 year
  - ▷ Significantly greater improvement in the exercise class group compared to:
    - ≫ Individual multimodal physiotherapy group ($P < 0.001$)
    - ≫ Home exercise group ($P < 0.001$)
  - ▷ Significant improvement in shoulder symptoms on Oxford and Constant scores ($P < 0.001$)
- ▶ Range of motion
  - ▷ Significant improvement from baseline in forward elevation and external rotation in all 3 groups
  - ▷ Significantly greater improvement in both of the physiotherapy intervention groups over the home exercise group at all time points ($P < 0.001$)
- ▶ Individual multimodal physiotherapy group showed significantly better Constant scores ($P = 0.002$) and Oxford scores ($P < 0.001$) than the home exercise group at all time points

- Hospital Anxiety and Disability Scale scores significantly improved during the course of treatment ($P < 0.001$)
  - ▷ The improvement in HADS anxiety score was significantly greater in both physiotherapy intervention groups than in home exercises alone.

Conclusions

- Hospital-based exercise class is more effective than individual physiotherapy or a home exercise program.
- Hospital-based exercise class can produce a rapid recovery from a frozen shoulder with a minimum number of hospital visits.

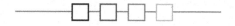

REVIEW ARTICLES

Neviaser RJ, Neviaser TJ. The frozen shoulder: diagnosis and management. *Clin Orthop*. 1987;223:59–64.

Warner JJ. Frozen shoulder: diagnosis and management. *J Am Acad Orthop Surg*. 1997;5:130–140.

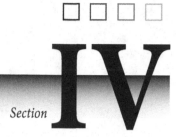

Section **IV**

Elbow

VI

Elbow

Lateral Epicondylitis

Chapter **24**

FEATURED ARTICLE

Authors: Bisset L, Beller E, Jull G, Brooks P, Darnell R, Vicenzino B.

Title: Mobilisation with movement and exercise, corticosteroid injection, or wait and see for tennis elbow: randomised trial.

Journal Information: *BMJ.* 2006;333:939.

Study Design: Prospective Randomized Study

▸ 198 patients with clinical diagnosis of tennis elbow and a minimum 6 weeks duration without any prior active treatment randomized to 1 of 3 treatments:
  ▷ Physiotherapy (8 sessions of elbow manipulation and exercise)
  ▷ Corticosteroid injection
  ▷ "Wait and see" approach
▸ Patients ages 18 to 65
▸ Main outcome measurements (measured at baseline, 3, 6, 12, 26, and 52 weeks)
  ▷ Global improvement (6-point Likert scale, with much improved and completely recovered graded as successes)
  ▷ Grip force (measured with a digital grip dynamometer)
  ▷ Assessor's rating of severity (symptoms rated by a blinded assessor using a visual analog score [VAS] scale 0 to 100)

Miller MD, Mauffrey C, Hak DJ.
Rapid Reference Review in Sports Medicine:
Pivotal Papers Revealed (pp 271-276).
© 2016 Taylor & Francis Group.

Results

▶ Corticosteroid injection group significantly better at 6 weeks but had a high later recurrence rate (47/65 of early successes subsequently regressed).

▶ Corticosteroid injection group had significantly poorer outcomes at 52 weeks compared to physiotherapy.

▶ Physiotherapy group was superior to wait-and-see group at 6 weeks.

▶ No difference between physiotherapy group and wait-and-see group at 52 weeks, when most participants in both groups reported a successful outcome.

▶ Physiotherapy treatment group sought less additional treatment, such as nonsteroidal anti-inflammatory drugs, than did those in the wait-and-see or injection groups.

Conclusions

▶ Physiotherapy combining elbow manipulation and exercise is superior to wait-and-see at 6 weeks and to corticosteroid injections after 6 weeks, providing a reasonable alternative to injections in the mid to long term.

▶ The significant short-term benefits of corticosteroid injection are reversed after 6 weeks with a high recurrence rate, implying that this treatment should be used with caution in the management of tennis elbow.

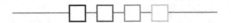

FEATURED ARTICLE

Authors: Haake M, König IR, Decker T, Riedel C, Buch M, Müller HH, Extracorporeal Shock Wave Therapy Clinical Trial Group.

Title: Extracorporeal shock wave therapy in the treatment of lateral epicondylitis: a randomized multicenter trial.

Journal Information: *J Bone Joint Surg Am.* 2002;84-A(11):1982–1991.

Study Design: Prospective Randomized Study

▶ Randomized multicenter trial with a parallel-group design

- Inclusion criteria:
  - ▷ At least 6 months of unsuccessful conservative therapy with ≥ 3 injections, ≥ 10 individual physiotherapy treatments, and ≥ 10 individual treatments with physical forms of therapy
  - ▷ ≥ 2-week interval since the last conservative therapy treatment
- Randomized to:
  - ▷ Extracorporeal shock wave therapy with 3 treatments of 2000 pulses each and a positive energy flux density (ED+) of 0.07 to 0.09 mJ/mm^2 (134 patients)
  - ▷ Placebo therapy (137 patients)
- Average patient age 46.6 years, 143 women, 128 men
- Average duration of symptoms 25 weeks
- Primary endpoints at 12 weeks
  - ▷ Success rate based on Roles and Maudsley pain score (score of 1 or 2 on 1 to 4 scale)
  - ▷ Whether additional treatment was required
- Crossover was possible after assessment of the primary end point
- Secondary end points at 6 and 12 weeks and 12 months
  - ▷ Roles and Maudsley pain score
  - ▷ Subjective pain rating (0- to 10-point scale)
  - ▷ Grip strength

Results

- No difference in primary end point at 12 weeks
  - ▷ 25.8% success rate in extracorporeal shock wave therapy group
  - ▷ 25.4% success rate in the placebo group
- No difference between groups in the secondary end points
- Improvement was seen in 2/3 of the patients in both groups at 12 months
- Few side effects were reported.

Conclusions

- Extracorporeal shock wave therapy as applied in the present study was ineffective in the treatment of lateral epicondylitis.
- Authors concluded that the previously reported success of extracorporeal shock wave therapy was attributable to inappropriate study designs.

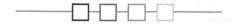

FEATURED ARTICLE

Authors: Nirschl RP, Pettrone FA.

Title: Tennis elbow. The surgical treatment of lateral epicondylitis.

Journal Information: *J Bone Joint Surg Am.* 1979;61:832–839.

A Top 100 Cited Articles in Clinical Orthopedic Sports Medicine

Study Design: Cohort Study

▶ 88 elbows in 82 patients out of 1213 clinical cases of lateral epicondylitis that failed to respond to conservative therapy

▶ These patients underwent a specific surgical technique that included exposure of the extensor carpi radialis brevis, excision of the identified lesion, and repair of the interface between the extensor carpi radialis longus and the anterior edge of the extensor aponeurosis with a running 0 chromic suture.

▶ 44 men, average age 45 years (30 to 63)

▶ 38 women, average age 41.5 years (27 to 58)

▶ Average follow-up 25 months (6 to 111 months)

▶ Average preop symptom duration 21.6 months (12 to 132 months) in men and 52 months (6 to 120 months) in women

▶ Grading system

▷ Excellent = full return to all activity with no pain

▷ Good = full return to all activity with occasional mild pain

▷ Fair = normal activity with no pain, significant pain with heavy activity, and 75% or better subjective overall improvement in pain

▷ Failure = no relief of preop symptoms

Results

▶ Immature fibroblastic and vascular infiltration of the origin of the extensor carpi radialis brevis was consistently identified at surgery.

▶ 87% responded to a post-op questionnaire, 46% had a follow-up examination, and remainder assessed by chart review.

▶ Outcome

▷ Excellent, 66 elbows

▷ Good, 9 elbows

▷ Fair, 11 elbows

▷ Failure, 2 elbows

- Overall rate of improvement 97.7%
- 85.2% returned to full activity, including rigorous sports
- 3 complications (2 infections, one mild loss of extension)

Conclusion

- The authors reported successful surgical outcomes for the surgical treatment of patients with lateral epicondylitis refractory to conservative therapy.

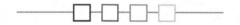

FEATURED ARTICLE

Authors: Regan W, Wold LE, Coonrad R, Morrey BF.

Title: Microscopic histopathology of chronic refractory lateral epicondylitis.

Journal Information: *Am J Sports Med.* 1992;20:746–749.

Study Design: Cohort Study

- Analyzed the histopathologic features from 11 patients treated surgically for lateral epicondylitis and compared to similar tissue from 12 cadaveric specimens
- Patients with epicondylitis were refractory to conservative treatment.
- Average age of surgical patients 40 years (19 to 56 years)
- Time from symptom onset to surgery averaged 26.2 months (7 to 96 months)

Results

- Macroscopic changes at the origin of the extensor carpi radialis brevis were observed in all surgical patients.
- 4/11 (36%) also had involvement of the common extensor origin.
- All 12 of the control specimens were reported as being without histologic abnormality.
- All 11 surgical specimens were interpreted as abnormal.
  ▷ Vascular proliferation was present in 10/11.
  ▷ Focal hyaline degeneration was recorded in all 11.
- Vascular proliferation and focal hyaline degeneration were not seen in any of the controls.

Conclusions

▶ The data suggest that chronic refractory lateral epicondylitis requiring surgery is a degenerative rather than inflammatory process.

▶ This may explain why anti-inflammatory medication is not successful treatment.

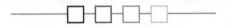

REVIEW ARTICLES

Ahmad Z, Siddiqui N, Malik SS, Abdus-Samee M, Tytherleigh-Strong G, Rushton N. Lateral epicondylitis: a review of pathology and management. *Bone Joint J*. 2013;95-B:1158–1164.

Calfee RP, Patel A, DaSilva MF, Akelman E. Management of lateral epicondylitis: current concepts. *J Am Acad Orthop Surg*. 2008;16:19–29.

□ □ □ □

Medial Epicondylitis

Chapter **25**

FEATURED ARTICLE

Authors: Stahl S, Kaufman T.

Title: The efficacy of an injection of steroids for medial epicondylitis. A prospective study of sixty elbows.

Journal Information: *J Bone Joint Surg.* 1997;79:1648–1652.

Study Design: Prospective Randomized Study

- Prospective, randomized, double-blind study of patients with medial epicondylitis who had not been previously managed with steroid injection
- 58 patients (60 elbows) randomized to either:
  - Single injection of 1% lidocaine with 40 mg of methylprednisolone (experimental group)
  - Saline solution (control group)
- Both groups were also managed with elimination of pain-producing activities, physical therapy, and the use of nonsteroidal anti-inflammatories.
- Similar mean age in both groups (43 years in control group, 41.3 years in experimental group)
- Both groups had similar gender, duration of the symptoms, degree of pain before injection, and number of dominant limbs involved.
- Outcome measurement
  - Pain assessment at 6 weeks, 3 months, and 1 year
  - Pain intensity (visual analog scale [VAS] 1 to 10)

Miller MD, Mauffrey C, Hak DJ.
Rapid Reference Review in Sports Medicine:
Pivotal Papers Revealed (pp 277-280).
© 2016 Taylor & Francis Group.

▷ Pain phase score: Modified the Nirschl and Pettrone grading system by adding another score to differentiate among varying intensities of pain during normal and strenuous activities

▷ 0 points = full activity and no pain

▷ 1 point = no pain during normal daily activities and mild pain during sports or occupational activity

▷ 2 points = occasional pain during normal daily activities and moderate pain during sports or occupational activity

▷ 3 points = mild to moderate pain during normal daily activities and severe pain during sports or occupational activity

▷ 4 points = pain at rest

Results

▸ At 6 weeks, the experimental group had significantly less pain than the control group ($P < 0.03$) on the pain phase score

▷ Average 1.2 ± 0.21 points in experimental group

▷ Average 1.9 ± 0.19 points in control group

▸ At 3 months and 1 year no difference between the 2 groups on the pain phase score

▸ Pain intensity (VAS) did not differ between the 2 groups at 6 weeks and 1 year

Conclusions

▸ The authors felt that the improvement observed in both groups primarily reflected the natural history of the disorder.

▸ Local steroid injections provide only short-term benefits in the treatment of medial epicondylitis.

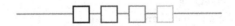

FEATURED ARTICLE

Authors: Vangsness CT Jr, Jobe FW.

Title: Surgical treatment of medial epicondylitis. Results in 35 elbows.

Journal Information: *J Bone Joint Surg Br.* 1991;73:409–411.

Study Design: Retrospective Review

▶ 35/38 consecutive patients who had operative treatment for medial epicondylitis after the failure of conservative management
▶ Mean duration of symptoms prior to surgery 22 months (5 to 48 months)
▶ Mean age 43 years (21 to 65 years), 32 men, 3 women
▶ Mean follow-up 85 months
▶ Although most cases of medial epicondylitis respond to conservative therapy, when conservative management fails and there is persistent pain after 6 to 12 months, surgical treatment must be considered.
▶ Surgical technique included detachment and reflection of the common flexor origin without disturbing the medial collateral ligament (MCL), excision of any abnormal tissue, placement of multiple drill holes in the medial epicondyle, and reattachment of the common flexor origin to this bleeding bone bed.
▶ Outcome measurements
  ▷ Nirschl and Pettrone grading system
  ▷ Excellent = full return to all activity with no pain
  ▷ Good = full return to all activity with occasional mild pain
  ▷ Fair = normal activity with no pain, significant pain with heavy activity, 75% or better overall improvement in pain
  ▷ Failure = no relief of preoperative symptoms

Results

▶ All patients had some improvement, and 86% of the patients had no limitation in the use of the elbow.
▶ Excellent 24 cases
▶ Good 10 cases
▶ Fair 1 case
▶ Residual tears with incomplete healing were consistently found in the flexor origin at the medial epicondyle, and microscopy showed reactive fibrous connective tissue with varying degrees of inflammation.

- Mean subjective estimate of elbow function improved from 38% to 98% of normal
- Isokinetic and grip strength testing in 16 patients showed no significant difference compared to the unoperated elbow.

Conclusion

- Surgery for failure of conservative treatment of medial epicondylitis is predictably efficacious in relieving pain, restoring strength, and allowing a return to the previous level of daily living and sports activity.

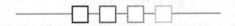

REVIEW ARTICLES

Ciccotti MC, Schwartz MA, Ciccotti MG. Diagnosis and treatment of medial epicondylitis of the elbow. *Clin Sports Med*. 2004;23:693–705.

Jobe JW, Ciccotti MG. Lateral and medial epicondylitis of the elbow. *J Am Acad Orthop Surg*. 1994;2:1–8.

Van Hofwegen C, Baker CL 3rd, Baker CL Jr. Epicondylitis in the athlete's elbow. *Clin Sports Med*. 2010;29:577–597.

□ □ □ □

Distal Biceps Rupture

Chapter **26**

FEATURED ARTICLE

Authors: Grewal R, Athwal GS, MacDermid JC, Faber KJ, Drosdowech DS, El-Hawary R, King GJ.

Title: Single versus double-incision technique for the repair of acute distal biceps tendon ruptures: a randomized clinical trial.

Journal Information: *J Bone Joint Surg Am.* 2012;94:1166–1174.

Study Design: Prospective Randomized Study

▶ Patients with acute distal biceps rupture randomized to:
  ▷ Single-incision repair with use of 2 suture anchors (n = 47)
  ▷ Double-incision repair with use of transosseous drill holes (n = 44)
▶ Outcome assessments at 3, 6, 12, and 24 months post-op
  ▷ Primary outcome measure
    ≫ American Shoulder and Elbow Surgeons (ASES) elbow score
  ▷ Secondary outcomes
    ≫ Muscle strength
    ≫ Complication rates
    ≫ Disabilities of the Arm, Shoulder and Hand (DASH) score
    ≫ Patient-Rated Elbow Evaluation (PREE) score
▶ Average age 45.1 years, all male

Miller MD, Mauffrey C, Hak DJ.
Rapid Reference Review in Sports Medicine:
Pivotal Papers Revealed (pp 281-286).
© 2016 Taylor & Francis Group.

- 79% (72/91) were followed for a minimum of 1 year with completion of both outcome questionnaires and clinical assessments for range of motion and strength.
- 91% (83/91) completed outcome questionnaires at 2 years.

Results

- No differences in the outcomes at 2 years between the 2 groups
- American Shoulder and Elbow Surgeons pain score ($P = 0.4$)
  - ▷ Single incision 4.6 ± 8.0
  - ▷ Double incision 4.4 ± 8.5
- American Shoulder and Elbow Surgeons function score ($P = 0.10$)
  - ▷ Single incision 32.6 ± 5.2
  - ▷ Double incision 34.6 ± 3.7
- Disabilities of the Arm, Shoulder and Hand score ($P = 0.3$)
  - ▷ Single incision 7.8 ± 12.9
  - ▷ Double incision 5.5 ± 11.8
- Patient-Rated Elbow Evaluation score ($P = 0.4$)
  - ▷ Single incision 6.1 ± 14.6
  - ▷ Double incision 4.9 ± 13.0
- No differences in isometric extension, pronation, or supination strength at > 1 year
- A 10% advantage in final isometric flexion strength was seen in the patients treated with the double-incision technique ($P = 0.01$).
  - ▷ Single incision 94%
  - ▷ Double incision 104%
- No differences in the rate of strength recovery
- Single-incision technique was associated with more early transient neurapraxias of the lateral antebrachial cutaneous nerve (19/47 vs 3/43, $p < 0.001$).
- 4 reruptures, all of which were related to patient noncompliance or reinjury during the early post-op period and appeared to be unrelated to the fixation technique ($P = 0.3$).

Conclusions

- The authors found no significant difference in outcomes between the single- and double-incision distal biceps repair techniques other than a 10% advantage in final flexion strength with the double-incision technique.
- Most complications were minor, with a significantly greater incidence in the single-incision group.

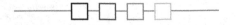

CLASSIC ARTICLE

Authors: Boyd JB, Anderson LD.

Title: A method for reinsertion of the distal biceps brachii tendon.

Journal Information: *J Bone Joint Surg.* 1961;43A:1041–1043.

▶ In this article the authors recommended a new method of distal biceps tendon insertion into the radial tuberosity.
▶ 2 advantages over other reported techniques:
  ▷ The tendon is replaced in its anatomic insertion with restoration of supination power.
  ▷ The replacement is accomplished with relative ease and without the difficulties and dangers inherent in the anterior approach.
▶ The authors reported that this method had been used in 3 patients at the Campbell Clinic with good results and without nerve damage or vascular complications.

Technique

▶ Curvilinear incision over the anterior aspect of the elbow
▶ Deep fascia is incised and the tendon of the biceps located
▶ Care is taken to protect the lateral antebrachial cutaneous nerve.
▶ A heavy silk suture is placed in the tendon with both ends emerging through the distal tip.
▶ Locate the opening of the canal, through which the tendon originally passed between the radius and the ulna, with a blunt instrument.
▶ Then flex the forearm and make a second incision over the posterolateral aspect of the elbow.
▶ Detach the muscles attached to the lateral surface of the olecranon and retract them laterally along the plane of the interosseous membrane to expose the head and neck of the radius.
▶ The deep branch of the radial nerve is not seen—it enters the forearm by winding around the neck of the radius between the planes of the supinator and is protected by the substance of this muscle when the supinator is retracted laterally.
▶ Fully pronate the forearm to expose the radial tuberosity.
▶ Make a trap in the radial tuberosity and place 2 drill holes opposite the hinge.
▶ Through the anterior incision, the ends of the suture previously placed in the biceps tendon are passed through the canal of the tendon using a tendon carrier or a hemostat.

▶ Traction on the suture pulls the tendon through the canal and into the posterior exposure.

▶ Thread the suture through the trap door and out the drill hole.

▶ The elbow is flexed to release tension on the tendon, the end of the tendon is placed in the trap door, and the suture is securely tied.

▶ A posterior splint is applied with the elbow flexed 10 degrees above a right angle and the forearm in moderate supination.

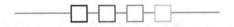

FEATURED ARTICLE

Authors: D'Alessandro DF, Shields CL Jr, Tibone JE, Chandler RW.

Title: Repair of distal biceps tendon ruptures in athletes.

Journal Information: *Am J Sports Med.* 1993;21:114–119.

Study Design: Retrospective Review

▶ 10/18 patients who underwent distal biceps tendon rupture between 1980 and 1989

▶ Average age 40 years (25 to 49), 10 men, 8 women

▶ 8 patients were weight lifters or body builders

▶ Surgical repair using double-incision technique

▶ Average follow-up 50 months (12 to 105 months)

▶ Evaluated by questionnaire, physical examination, and radiographs to determine their functional recovery

▷ 8 patients also evaluated by isokinetic muscle testing in supination and flexion

Results

▶ Patients uniformly graded their subjective results as excellent (mean rating 9.75/10).

▶ All athletes returned to full, unlimited activity.

▶ The contour of the biceps muscle was restored in all cases.

▶ Isokinetic muscle testing

▷ Repaired dominant extremities

» Supination strength and endurance were normal.
» Flexion strength normal, but averaged 20% less endurance
▷ Repaired nondominant extremities
» Supination strength deficit of 25%, but normal endurance
» Flexion strength and endurance were normal.

Conclusions

▶ The authors concluded that anatomic repair of a distal biceps tendon rupture gives consistently excellent subjective and good objective results in athletes, especially those with high strength demands such as weight lifting and body building.

▶ The authors emphasized the importance of rehabilitation of the operated arm, especially the repaired nondominant extremity.

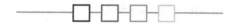

FEATURED ARTICLE

Authors: Baker BE, Bierwagen D.

Title: Rupture of the distal tendon of the biceps brachii. Operative versus non-operative treatment.

Journal Information: *J Bone Joint Surg Am*. 1985;67:414–417.

Study Design: Retrospective Review

▶ 13 patients sustaining distal biceps rupture
▷ 10 treated operatively with a 2-incision technique
▷ 3 treated nonoperatively
▶ Average age 49 years (33 to 67 years), all men
▶ Cybex isokinetic dynamometer testing performed 15 months to 6 years after injury
▶ Cybex isokinetic dynamometer testing also performed on 10 normal men (age range 19 to 47 years)

Results

▶ Injuries that underwent surgical repair showed a return to normal levels of strength and endurance of both elbow flexion and forearm supination.

- ▶ Injuries that were treated nonoperatively had a remaining deficit in strength and endurance of both elbow flexion and forearm supination.
  - ▷ All 3 complained of weakness of supination power, particularly in performing functions such as using a screwdriver or hammer.
- ▶ Normal controls
  - ▷ Compared to their nondominant arm, their dominant arm had:
    - » 27% greater supination strength
    - » 39% greater supination endurance
    - » 15% greater elbow flexion strength
    - » 41% greater elbow flexion endurance
- ▶ Operative treatment
  - ▷ Compared to their uninjured arm, their repaired arm had:
    - » 13% greater supination strength
    - » 32% greater supination endurance
    - » 9% greater elbow flexion strength
    - » 9% greater elbow flexion endurance
- ▶ Nonoperative treatment
  - ▷ Compared to their uninjured arm, their injured arm had:
    - » 27% less supination strength
    - » 47% less supination endurance
    - » 21% less elbow flexion strength
    - » 21% less elbow flexion endurance

Conclusions

- ▶ Patients with distal biceps tendon ruptures treated nonoperatively can expect weakness in strength and endurance of both flexion and supination.
- ▶ The 2-incision technique for distal biceps tendon repair appears to be safe and effective in restoring function.

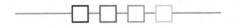

REVIEW ARTICLES

Ramsey ML. Distal biceps tendon injuries: diagnosis and management. *J Am Acad Orthop Surg*. 1999;7:199–207.

Sutton KM, Dodds SD, Ahmad CS, Sethi PM. Surgical treatment of distal biceps rupture. J *Am Acad Orthop Surg*. 2010;18:139–148.

Throwing Injuries

Chapter 27

CLASSIC ARTICLE

Authors: Jobe FW, Stark H, Lombardo SJ.

Title: Reconstruction of the ulnar collateral ligament in athletes.

Journal Information: *J Bone Joint Surg Am.* 1986;68:1158–1163.

Study Design: Retrospective Review

▶ Details the operative repair now referred to as Tommy John surgery

▶ Tommy John, a pitcher for the Los Angeles Dodgers, was the first patient to undergo this procedure in 1974. He missed the 1975 season rehabilitating his arm before returning for the 1976 season, and following his return he went on to win 164 games, retiring in 1989.

▶ Retrospective review of 16 athletes who underwent ulnar collateral ligament reconstruction using a free tendon graft for valgus instability

▶ Ages 20 to 31, all men

▶ 12 were professional baseball pitchers, 1 college baseball pitcher, 1 professional centerfielder, 2 javelin throwers

Operative Procedure

▶ Anterior portion of the ulnar collateral ligament exposed

▶ Common flexor bundle and most of the pronator teres were elevated by transection of the tendon, leaving a fringe of tendon on the epicondyle for reattachment.

Miller MD, Mauffrey C, Hak DJ.
*Rapid Reference Review in Sports Medicine:
Pivotal Papers Revealed (pp 287-294).*
© 2016 Taylor & Francis Group.

▶ The ulnar nerve was mobilized and protected.

▶ Any calcifications or bony particles were removed from the ligament and the surrounding soft tissue.

▶ 3.2-mm drill holes placed in the medial epicondyle and ulna, corresponding to the points of attachment of the torn ligament

▶ A donor tendon was passed through the holes in a figure-of-8 pattern.

▷ Palmaris longus (12 patients)

▷ Plantaris (3 patients)

▷ Achilles tendon strip 3 mm wide and 15 cm long (1 patient)

▶ Graft was pulled taut and sutured to itself

▶ Ulnar nerve transferred anterior to the medial epicondyle

▶ Arm immobilized with a posterior splint

Results

▶ 10/16 patients returned to their previous level of participation in sports.

▶ 1/16 returned to a lower level of participation.

▶ 5/16 retired from professional athletics, but "not as a result of the surgical procedure."

▶ 7 patients had returned to full activity by 1 year; the others returned by 18 months.

▶ Complications/reoperations

▷ 1 superficial post-op infection that resolved in 2 weeks

▷ High incidence of complications related to the ulnar nerve despite precautions

▷ 2 patients had post-op ulnar neuropathy (1 late, 1 early) that required a secondary operation, but they eventually recovered completely.

▷ 3 patients reported some transient post-op hypoesthesia along the ulnar aspect of the forearm that resolved after a few weeks or months.

▷ 1 college baseball pitcher had pain in the elbow when he resumed pitching. Nine months later he underwent reoperation for medial epicondylitis, removal of scar tissue from the ulnar nerve, and reattachment of the flexor muscles. He subsequently returned to pitching.

▷ 1 patient had a bone spur removed from his olecranon 7 months after the reconstruction.

Conclusions

▶ The authors postulate that the surgical reconstruction technique provides reconstitution of the ligament through slow graft revascularization.

▶ Interval from operation to effective pitching ranged from 11 to 19 months

▸ The authors allowed a few athletes to return to professional play 12 months post-op, but they were not permitted to participate at a full level until 18 months post-op.

▸ Athletes' strength and performance consistently improved during the second post-op year.

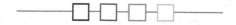

FEATURED ARTICLE

Authors: Osbahr DC, Cain EL Jr, Raines BT, Fortenbaugh D, Dugas JR, Andrews JR.

Title: Long-term outcomes after ulnar collateral ligament reconstruction in competitive baseball players: minimum 10-year follow-up.

Journal Information: *Am J Sports Med.* 2014;42:1333–1342.

2013 AAOSM O'Donoghue Award Winner

Study Design: Cohort Study

▸ Case series review of ulnar collateral ligament reconstructions (UCLR) performed on competitive baseball players with a minimum 10-year follow-up

▸ Surgical data were prospectively collected.

▸ Average age at surgery 22.1 years (15.9 to 41.7 years)

▸ Patients were surveyed by telephone follow-up, during which scoring systems were used to assess baseball career and post–baseball career outcomes.

 ▷ Modified Conway scale, which numerically ranks outcomes based on the highest post-operative level of competition compared with their level of competition at the time of surgery

 ▷ Disabilities of the Arm, Shoulder, and Hand (DASH)

▸ 256/313 (82%) patients were contacted.

 ▷ 228 (89%) were pitchers and 28 (11%) were position players.

 ▷ 24 were Major League Baseball players.

 ▷ 88 were Minor League Baseball players.

 ▷ 104 were collegiate baseball players.

 ▷ 40 were high school baseball players.

▶ Average time from surgery 12.6 years (range 10.1 to 17.1 years)

Results

▶ 49 players (19%) required a total of 59 additional surgeries after the primary UCLR.

▶ Overall, 83% were able to return to the same or higher level of competition in less than 1 year.

▶ 90% of these pitchers were able to return to the same or higher level of competition in less than 1 year.

▶ Baseball career longevity averaged 3.6 years in general and 2.9 years at the same or higher level of play.

▶ Major and Minor League players returned for longer than did collegiate and high school players after surgery ($P < 0.001$).

▷ Major League players 7.5 years ± 3.4 years

▷ Minor League players 4.2 years ± 3.5 years

▷ Collegiate players 2.5 years ± 1.9 years

▷ High school players 2.9 years ± 2.8 years

▶ At a minimum of 10-year follow-up, 243 (95%) of the baseball players were retired and 13 (5%) were still active in competitive baseball.

▶ Baseball retirement typically occurred for reasons other than elbow problems (86%).

▶ Many players had shoulder problems (34%) or shoulder surgery (25%) during their baseball career, which often resulted in retirement attributable to shoulder problems ($P < 0.001$).

▶ For post–baseball career outcomes, 92% of patients were able to throw without pain, and 98% were still able to participate in throwing at least on a recreational level.

▶ The 10-year minimum follow-up scores

▷ Disabilities of the Arm, Shoulder, and Hand overall 0.80 ± 4.43

▷ Disabilities of the Arm, Shoulder, and Hand work module 1.10 ± 6.90

▷ Disabilities of the Arm, Shoulder, and Hand sports module 2.88 ± 11.91

▶ 93% of patients were satisfied overall.

▶ 3% of patients reported persistent elbow pain.

▶ 5% of patients reported limitation of elbow function.

Conclusions

▶ At a minimum 10-year follow-up, most baseball players who had undergone UCLR were satisfied, with very few reporting persistent elbow pain or functional limitation.

▶ Most baseball players were able to return to the same or higher level of competition in less than 1 year with acceptable career longevity.

▸ Retirement from baseball was typically for reasons other than the elbow.

▸ Patients had excellent DASH score results for daily work and sporting activities.

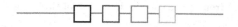

FEATURED ARTICLE

Authors: Cain EL Jr, Andrews JR, Dugas JR, Wilk KE, McMichael CS, Walter JC 2nd, Riley RS, Arthur ST.

Title: Outcome of ulnar collateral ligament reconstruction of the elbow in 1281 athletes: results in 743 athletes with minimum 2-year follow-up.

Journal Information: *Am J Sports Med.* 2010;38:2426–2434.

Study Design: Cohort Study

▸ Case series review of 1266 ulnar collateral reconstructions and 15 repairs performed in 1281 patients from 1988 to 2006 by a single surgeon

▸ Average age 21.5 years (14 to 59 years), 1253 men, 28 women

▸ 95% of injuries were from participating in baseball.

▸ Data were collected prospectively, and patients were surveyed retrospectively with a telephone questionnaire to determine outcomes and return to performance at a minimum of 2 years after surgery.

▸ Average follow-up 38.4 months (24 to 130 months)

▸ 942 patients had a minimum 2-year follow-up.

▸ 743 patients (79%) were contacted for follow-up evaluation and/or completed a questionnaire at an average of 37 months post-operatively.

  ▷ 596 (80%) had a phone interview.

  ▷ 147 (20%) were examined and completed a questionnaire during an office visit.

  ▷ 199 patients could not be contacted for evaluation and questionnaire.

Results

▸ 617 patients (83%) returned to the previous level of competition or higher.

  ▷ 610 after reconstruction

  ▷ 7 after repair

- Major League Baseball players
  - ▷ 34/45 (75.5%) returned to the same level.
  - ▷ 7 returned to the Minor League level.
  - ▷ 4 did not return to the sport.
- Average time from surgery to the initiation of throwing 4.4 months (2.8 to 12 months)
- Average time from surgery to full competition 11.6 months (3 to 72 months)
- Complications
  - ▷ 148 patients (20%) sustained a complication.
  - ▷ 80% (121 patients) of the complications were post-op ulnar nerve neurapraxia, most of which involved only sensory paresthesias that resolved within 6 weeks.

Conclusion

- Ulnar collateral ligament reconstruction with subcutaneous ulnar nerve transposition was found to be effective in correcting valgus elbow instability in the overhead athlete and allowed most athletes (83%) to return to previous or higher level of competition in less than 1 year.

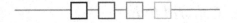

FEATURED ARTICLE

Authors: Conway JE, Jobe FW, Glousman RE, Pink M.

Title: Medial instability of the elbow in throwing athletes. Treatment by repair or reconstruction of the ulnar collateral ligament.

Journal Information: *J Bone Joint Surg Am*. 1992;74:67–83.

Study Design: Retrospective Review

- This later follow-up study expands on Jobe's original report (Jobe FW, Stark H, Lombardo SJ. Reconstruction of the ulnar collateral ligament in athletes. *J Bone Joint Surg Am*. 1986;68:1158-1163).
- Retrospective review of 71 patients with valgus elbow instability who underwent operative treatment from 1974 to 1987
- 71 patients
- 68 patients (70 operations) had > 2-year follow-up.

- ▶ Average follow-up 6.3 years (2 to 15 years)
- ▶ 14 patients had a direct repair of the incompetent ulnar collateral ligament.
- ▶ 56 patients had reconstruction using a free tendon graft.

Results

- ▶ Repair group (14 patients)
  - ▷ 10 excellent or good result
  - ▷ 7 returned to the previous level of participation in their sport.
  - ▷ 2/7 Major League Baseball players who had a repair as the primary operation (no previous operation on the elbow) returned to playing Major League baseball.
- ▶ Reconstruction group (56 patients)
  - ▷ 45 (80%) excellent or good result
  - ▷ 38 (68%) returned to the previous level of participation in their sport.
  - ▷ 12/16 Major League Baseball players who had a reconstruction as the primary operation (no previous operation on the elbow) returned to playing Major League baseball.
- ▶ 74% of patients in the reconstruction group returned to previous level of competition compared to 50% in the repair group, but this difference was not significant (chi-square test with Yates' correction, $P = 0.16$).
- ▶ Of the 27 Major League players, excellent results were obtained in 2/7 (29%) in the repair group and in 13/20 (65%) in the reconstruction group, but this difference was not significant (chi-square test with Yates' correction, $P = 0.22$).
- ▶ Previous operations on the elbow decreased the chance of returning to the previous level of sports participation ($P = 0.04$).
  - ▷ None of members of the repair group had undergone a prior operation.
  - ▷ 47 patients in the reconstruction group had no prior operations.
    - ≫ 35 (74%) excellent result
    - ≫ 39 (83%) excellent or good result
  - ▷ 9 patients in the reconstruction group had a prior operation.
    - ≫ 3 (33%) excellent result
    - ≫ 5 (55%) excellent or good result
- ▶ Complications
  - ▷ 15 patients (21%) had post-op ulnar neuropathy despite meticulous handling and transposition of the nerve.
  - ▷ 6 of these were transient, and 5 of these patients returned to previous level of sport
  - ▷ 9 patients had an additional operation for treatment of the neuropathy, and 4 of these patients returned to previous level of sport

▷ 4/6 patients who had a flexion deformity of 10 to 25 degrees after reconstruction still had an excellent functional result.

Conclusions

▶ Most athletes who had been unable to participate in throwing sports because of medial elbow instability were able to return to their previous level of participation after reconstruction of the anterior band of the ulnar collateral ligament with an autologous tendon graft.

▶ The chance of return to competitive sports was significantly reduced when prior operations had been performed on the elbow before reconstruction.

▶ Function of the ulnar nerve should be carefully assessed before the operation because of the possibility of post-op ulnar neuropathy.

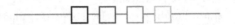

REVIEW ARTICLES

Bruce JR, Andrews JR. Ulnar collateral ligament injuries in the throwing athlete. *J Am Acad Orthop Surg.* 2014;22:315–325.

Dugas J, Chronister J, Cain EL Jr, Andrews JR. Ulnar collateral ligament in the overhead athlete: a current review. *Sports Med Arthrosc.* 2014;22:169–182.

Kinsella SD, Thomas SJ, Huffman GR, Kelly JD 4th. The thrower's shoulder. *Orthop Clin North Am.* 2014;45:387–401.

Loftice J, Fleisig GS, Zheng N, Andrews JR. Biomechanics of the elbow in sports. *Clin Sports Med.* 2004;23:519–530.

Maloney MD, Mohr KJ, el Attrache NS. Elbow injuries in the throwing athlete. Difficult diagnoses and surgical complications. *Clin Sports Med.* 1999;18:795–809.

Wilk KE, Meister K, Andrew JR. Current concepts in the rehabilitation of the overhead throwing athlete. *Am J Sports Med.* 2002;30:136–151.

Little Leaguer's Elbow

Chapter 28

FEATURED ARTICLE
Authors: Fleisig GS, Andrews JR, Cutter GR, Weber A, Loftice J, McMichael C, et al.
Title: Risk of serious injury for young baseball pitchers: a 10-year prospective study.
Journal Information: *Am J Sports Med.* 2011;39:253–257.

Study Design: Cohort Study

▸ Prospective cohort study of 481 youth pitchers (ages 9 to 14 years)

▸ Purpose: To quantify the cumulative incidence of throwing injuries in young baseball pitchers

▸ Participants interviewed annually for a total of 10 years

▸ Injury defined as elbow surgery, shoulder surgery, or retirement due to throwing injury

▸ Compared risk of injury between participants who pitched at least 4 years with those who pitched less

▸ Examined risk of injury for:

  ▷ Pitching > 100 innings in at least 1 calendar year

  ▷ Starting curveballs before age 13 years

  ▷ Playing catcher for at least 3 years

Results

▶ Cumulative incidence of injury was 5.0%

▶ Participants who pitched > 100 innings in a year were 3.5 times more likely to be injured (95% confidence interval = 1.16 to 10.44).

▶ Pitchers who concomitantly played catcher seemed to be injured more frequently, but this trend was not significant with the study sample size.

Conclusions

▶ The risk of a youth pitcher sustaining a serious throwing injury within 10 years is 5%

▶ Pitching > 100 innings in 1 year significantly increases risk of injury.

▶ Limiting the number of innings pitched per year may reduce the risk of injury.

▶ The study was unable to demonstrate that curveballs before age 13 increase risk of injury.

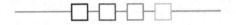

FEATURED ARTICLE

Authors: Lyman S, Fleisig GS, Andrews JR, Osinski ED.

Title: Effect of pitch type, pitch count, and pitching mechanics on risk of elbow and shoulder pain in youth baseball pitchers.

Journal Information: *Am J Sports Med.* 2002;30:463–468.

Study Design: Cohort Study

▶ Prospective cohort study of 476 Little League Baseball pitchers (ages 9 to 14 years) followed for one season to evaluate the association between pitch counts, pitch types, and pitching mechanics and shoulder and elbow pain

▶ Data sources
  ▷ Preseason and postseason questionnaires
  ▷ Performance interviews after each game
  ▷ Pitch count logs
  ▷ Video analysis of pitching mechanics

Results

▶ 50% of pitchers experienced elbow or shoulder pain during the season.

▶ 28% experienced elbow pain at least once during the season.

▶ About 7% of all pitching appearances resulted in elbow pain.

▶ 35% experienced shoulder pain at least once during the season.

▶ More than 9% of all pitching appearances resulted in shoulder pain.

▶ Overall, almost 15% of all pitching appearances resulted in either elbow or shoulder pain.

▶ Curveball was associated with a 52% increased risk of shoulder pain

▶ Slider was associated with an 86% increased risk of elbow pain

▶ Significant association between the number of pitches thrown in a game and during the season and the rate of elbow pain and shoulder pain

Conclusions

▶ Pitchers in this age group should be cautioned about throwing breaking pitches (curveballs and sliders) because of the increased risk of elbow and shoulder pain.

▶ Limitations on pitches thrown in a game and in a season can also reduce the risk of pain.

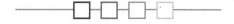

REVIEW ARTICLES

Benjamin HJ, Briner WW Jr. Little League elbow. *Clin J Sport Med.* 2005;15:37–40.

Congeni J. Treating and preventing Little League elbow. *Phys Sports Med.* 1994;22:54–64.

Hutchinson MR, Wynn S. Biomechanics and development of the elbow in the young throwing athlete. *Clin Sports Med.* 2004;23:531–544, viii.

Stanitski CL. Combating overuse injuries: a focus on children and adolescents. *Phys Sports Med.* 1993;21:87–106.

Osteochondritis Dissecans of the Capitellum

Chapter 29

FEATURED ARTICLE

Authors: Takahara M, Mura N, Sasaki J, Harada M, Ogino T.

Title: Classification, treatment, and outcome of osteochondritis dissecans of the humeral capitellum.

Journal Information: *J Bone Joint Surg Am.* 2007;89:1205–1214.

Study Design: Retrospective Review

- ▶ 106 patients with osteochondritis dissecans of the capitellum
- ▶ Average age at time of initial presentation 15.3 years (10 to 34 years)
- ▶ Capitellar growth plate was open in 18 patients and closed in 88
- ▶ 36 patients treated nonoperatively
- ▶ 70 patients treated operatively
  - ▷ 55 underwent fragment removal alone.
  - ▷ 12 underwent fragment fixation with a bone graft.
  - ▷ 3 underwent reconstruction of the articular surface with use of osteochondral plug grafts from the lateral femoral condyle.
- ▶ Average follow-up 7.2 years (6 months to 25 years)
- ▶ Outcome assessments
  - ▷ Pain
    - » None
    - » Mild (pain only after intense activity, such as sports or work)
    - » Moderate or severe (pain after daily activities or even at rest)

Miller MD, Mauffrey C, Hak DJ.
Rapid Reference Review in Sports Medicine:
Pivotal Papers Revealed (pp 299-303).
© 2016 Taylor & Francis Group.

▷ Return to sports
  » Competitive (a complete return)
  » Recreational (an incomplete return)
  » Substantial limitation (a change or cessation of the sport)
▷ Radiographic findings

Results

▸ Patients with an open capitellar physis and a good elbow range of motion had good outcomes.
▸ Continued elbow stress resulted in the worst outcome in terms of pain and radiographic findings.
▸ Surgery provided significantly better results than elbow rest ($P < 0.01$) in patients with a closed capitellar physis.
▸ Fragment fixation or reconstruction provided significantly better results than fragment removal alone ($P < 0.05$).
▸ Results of removal alone were dependent on the size of the defect in the capitellum.
▸ Outcome in terms of pain was closely associated with sports activity and radiographic findings.

Conclusions

▸ The authors concluded that osteochondritis dissecans of the capitellum can be classified as stable or unstable.
▸ Stable lesions that healed completely with elbow rest had all of the following findings at the time of the initial presentation:
  ▷ Open capitellar growth plate
  ▷ Localized flattening or radiolucency of the subchondral bone
  ▷ Good elbow motion
▸ Unstable lesions, for which surgery provided significantly better results, had one of the following findings:
  ▷ Closed capitellar growth plate
  ▷ Fragmentation
  ▷ Restriction of elbow motion of ≥ 20 degrees
▸ Fragment fixation or reconstruction of the articular surface leads to better results than simple excision in large unstable lesions.

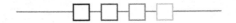

FEATURED ARTICLE

Authors: Mihara K, Suzuki K, Makuichi D, Nishinaka N, Yamaguchi K, Tsutsui H.

Title: Surgical treatment for osteochondritis dissecans of the humeral capitellum.

Journal Information: *J Shoulder Elbow Surg.* 2010;19:31–37.

Study Design: Retrospective Review

- 27 patients with advanced osteochondritis dissecans lesions of the capitellus treated operatively
- Mean age at surgery 13.3 years (10 to 16 years), all male baseball players
- Mean time from symptoms onset to initial presentation 8.1 months (1 to 36 months)
- Mean time from initial presentation to operation 3.6 months (2 weeks to 17 months)
- Surgery recommended if fragment unstable or loose body seen on radiographs and/or magnetic resonance imaging and/or an episode of locking (23 patients met these criteria)
- In 4 patients, the lesion deteriorated radiographically during initial conservative treatment of an early osteochondritis dissecans lesion, and surgery was then recommended.
- Surgical treatment
  - ▷ Drilling to the lesion (3 patients)
  - ▷ Fragment fixation with the bone-peg graft and/or resorbable pin (7 patients)
  - ▷ Pull-out wiring (6 patients)
  - ▷ Removal of the detached fragment with drilling (4 patients)
  - ▷ Articular surface using an osteochondral rib autograft (7 patients)
- Mean follow-up 37.4 months (24 to 92 months)
- Outcome assessment
  - ▷ Modified elbow rating system
    - » Subjective score
      - ⟩ Pain
      - ⟩ Swelling
      - ⟩ Locking
      - ⟩ Sports activity

>> Objective score
> Flexion contracture
> Pronation/supination range of motion
> Sagittal arc of motion
>> Excellent (90 to 100)
>> Good (90 to 89)
>> Fair (60 to 79)
>> Poor (< 60)
▷ Radiographic evaluation
▷ Return to sports.

Results

▶ Significant improvement in mean subjective elbow score ($P < 0.0001$)
  ▷ 70 preop
  ▷ 96 at follow-up
▶ Significant improvement in mean objective elbow score ($P = 0.0176$)
  ▷ 71 preop
  ▷ 81 at follow-up
▶ 25 patients returned to baseball post-operatively.
▶ No patients reported a decrease in baseball performance level compared to that at their initial presentation.
▶ Final follow-up radiographs
  ▷ 4 had flattening of > 70% of the capitellum or degenerative changes.
  ▷ 3 of these patients had undergone fragment removal, and one had failure of fragment reattachment.
  ▷ Remodeling of the capitellar lateral margin was insufficient in these 4 patients.

Conclusions

▶ Surgical treatment was useful to restore advanced osteochondritis dissecans lesions.
▶ Authors concluded that reconstruction of the capitellar lateral margin is important for achieving good clinical results.

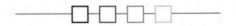

REVIEW ARTICLES

Bradley JP, Petrie RS. Osteochondritis dissecans of the humeral capitellum. Diagnosis and treatment. *Clin Sports Med.* 2001;20:565–590.

Ruchelsman DE, Hall MP, Youm T. Osteochondritis dissecans of the capitellum: current concepts. *J Am Acad Orthop Surg.* 2010;18:557–567.

Schenck RC Jr, Goodnight JM. Current concepts review: osteochondritis dissecans. *J Bone Joint Surg Am.* 1996;78:439–456.

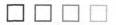

Miscellaneous Elbow Topics

Chapter **30**

FEATURED ARTICLE

Authors: O'Driscoll SW, Bell DF, Morrey BF.

Title: Posterolateral rotatory instability of the elbow.

Journal Information: *J Bone Joint Surg Am.* 1991;73:440–446.

A Top 100 Cited Articles in Clinical Orthopedic Sports Medicine

- Authors' first description of recurrent posterolateral rotatory instability of the elbow
- Reported on their treatment of 5 patients, ages 5 to 46 years, 3 males, 2 females
- Patients complain of mechanical symptoms (clicking, catching, etc) with elbow extension
- Caused by laxity of the ulnar part of the lateral collateral ligament (LCL)
  - Transient rotatory subluxation of the ulnohumeral joint
  - Secondary dislocation of the radiohumeral joint
  - Annular ligament is intact so the radioulnar joint does not dislocate.

Results

- Treated by operative repair of the lax ulnar part of the LCL
- Instability demonstrated by posterolateral rotatory-instability test
  - Forearm is supinated; valgus and axial compression is applied to the elbow while it is flexed from full extension

Miller MD, Mauffrey C, Hak DJ.
Rapid Reference Review in Sports Medicine:
Pivotal Papers Revealed (pp 305-306).
© 2016 Taylor & Francis Group.

▷ In full extension elbow is reduced; as the elbow is flexed to 20 to 30 degrees, the radiohumeral joint subluxes; further flexion to about 40 degrees produces a sudden palpable and visible reduction of the radiohumeral joint

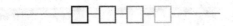

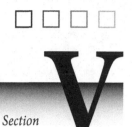

Ankle

□ □ □ □

Ankle Sprains

Chapter **31**

FEATURED ARTICLE

Authors: Pihlajamäki H, Hietaniemi K, Paavola M, Visuri T, Mattila VM.

Title: Surgical versus functional treatment for acute ruptures of the lateral ligament complex of the ankle in young men: a randomized controlled trial.

Journal Information: *J Bone Joint Surg Am.* 2010 ;92:2367–2374.

Study Design: Prospective Randomized Study

- Long-term follow-up of a prospective randomized study of Finnish military men sustaining an acute grade III lateral ankle ligament rupture
  - Surgical treatment (25 patients)
    - Suture repair of injured ligament(s) within 1 week of injury, then short leg cast × 6 weeks, full weight bearing
  - Functional treatment (26 patients)
    - Aircast ankle brace × 3 weeks
- Average age 20.4 years (18 to 26 years), all men
- Outcome measurements
  - Final follow-up exam
  - Performance test protocol and scoring scale for the evaluation of ankle injuries

Miller MD, Mauffrey C, Hak DJ.
*Rapid Reference Review in Sports Medicine:
Pivotal Papers Revealed (pp 309-314).*
© 2016 Taylor & Francis Group.

▷ Stress radiographs

▷ Magnetic resonance imaging (MRI)

▶ 60% (15/25) of surgically treated patients and 69% (18/26) of functionally treated patients returned for long-term follow-up.

▶ Mean follow-up 14 years

Results

▶ All patients in both groups had recovered their preinjury activity level and reported that they could walk and run normally.

▶ Reinjury prevalence (risk difference: 32%; 95% confidence interval: 6% to 58%)

▷ 1/15 in the surgical group

▷ 7/18 in the functional treatment group

▶ Mean ankle score

▷ No significant difference between the groups

▶ Stress radiographs

▷ No difference in mean anterior drawer

» −1 mm in the surgical group

» 0 mm in the functional treatment group

▷ No difference in the mean talar tilt

» Zero degrees in both groups

▶ Magnetic resonance imaging

▷ Grade II osteoarthritis in 4/15 surgically treated patients

▷ No osteoarthritis in the 18 functionally treated patients

Conclusions

▶ In terms of recovery of the preinjury activity level, the long-term results of surgical treatment of acute lateral ligament rupture of the ankle is comparable to that of functional treatment.

▶ Surgical treatment appeared to decrease the prevalence of reinjury of the lateral ligaments, but may increase the risk for subsequent development of osteoarthritis.

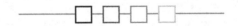

FEATURED ARTICLE

Authors: Beynnon BD, Renström PA, Haugh L, Uh BS, Barker H.

Title: A prospective, randomized clinical investigation of the treatment of first-time ankle sprains.

Journal Information: *Am J Sports Med.* 2006;34:1401–1412.

Study Design: Prospective Randomized Trial

▸ Patients suffering their first ligament ankle injury were stratified by the severity of the sprain (grades I, II, or III) and then randomized to undergo functional treatment with different types of external supports.

▸ Patients completed daily logs until they returned to normal function and were followed up at 6 months.

▸ Primary outcome measures

▷ Time required to return to normal (preinjury) walking

▷ Time required to return to normal (preinjury) stair climbing

▷ Time required to place full weight on the ankle without a limp

▸ Secondary outcomes

▷ Time required to return to full weight bearing

▷ Time to experience no pain during full weight bearing

▷ Time to obtain full function in normal activities of daily living

▷ Time to return to full capability in work or school activity

▷ Time to return to full capability in usual athletic or recreational activity

▸ During the study period, 130 patients completed the baseline, primary/secondary outcome response, and tertiary outcomes obtained at 6 months follow-up.

▷ 44 grade I sprains

▷ 68 grade II sprains

▷ 18 grade III sprains

Results

▸ Grade I sprains treated with the Air-Stirrup brace combined with an elastic wrap returned to normal walking ($P = 0.0008$) and stair climbing ($P = 0.003$) in half the time compared to the Air-Stirrup brace alone or the elastic wrap alone.

- ▷ Air-Stirrup combined with elastic wrap
  - » Mean 4.62 days to return to normal walking
  - » Mean 5.46 days to return to normal stair climbing
- ▷ Elastic wrap alone
  - » Mean 11.6 days to return to normal walking
  - » Mean 12.05 days to return to normal stair climbing
- ▷ Air-Stirrup brace alone
  - » Mean 10.33 days to return to normal walking
  - » Mean 11.43 days to return to normal stair climbing
- ▶ Grade II sprains with the Air-Stirrup brace combined with the elastic wrap returned to normal walking ($P = 0.0001$) and stair climbing ($P = 0.0001$) significantly faster than with cast immobilization for 10 days followed by bracing.
  - ▷ Air-Stirrup combined with elastic wrap
    - » Mean 10.1 days to return to normal walking
    - » Mean 11.72 days to return to normal stair climbing
  - ▷ Elastic wrap alone
    - » Mean 11.67 days to return to normal walking
    - » Mean 13.38 days to return to normal stair climbing
  - ▷ Air-Stirrup brace alone
    - » Mean 13.38 days to return to normal walking
    - » Mean 16.38 days to return to normal stair climbing
  - ▷ Cast immobilization for 10 days followed by bracing
    - » Mean 24.12 days to return to normal walking
    - » Mean 27.94 days to return to normal stair climbing
- ▶ Grade III sprains had no difference between treatment with an Air-Stirrup brace or cast immobilization for 10 days followed by bracing.
  - ▷ Air-Stirrup combined with elastic wrap
    - » Mean 18.56 days to return to normal walking
    - » Mean 18.31 days to return to normal stair climbing
  - ▷ Cast immobilization for 10 days followed by bracing
    - » Mean 19 days to return to normal walking
    - » Mean 21.08 days to return to normal stair climbing
- ▶ The 6-month follow-up of each sprain severity group revealed no difference between the treatments for frequency of reinjury, ankle motion, and function.

Conclusion

▶ Treatment of first-time grade I and II ankle ligament sprains with the Air-Stirrup brace combined with an elastic wrap provides earlier return to preinjury function compared to use of the Air-Stirrup brace alone, an elastic wrap alone, or a walking cast for 10 days.

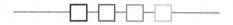

FEATURED ARTICLE

Authors: Boyce SH, Quigley MA, Campbell S.

Title: Management of ankle sprains: a randomised controlled trial of the treatment of inversion injuries using an elastic support bandage or an Aircast ankle brace.

Journal Information: *Br J Sports Med.* 2005;39:91–96.

Study Design: Prospective Randomized Trial

▶ 50 patients sustaining an ankle sprain randomized to:
  ▷ Elastic support bandage (17/25 completed the study)
  ▷ Aircast ankle brace (18/25 completed the study)
▶ Average age 32.2 years (16 to 58 years), 29 men, 21 women
▶ Follow-up at 2 to 3 days, 10 days, 1 month
▶ Primary outcome measure
  ▷ Ankle joint function at 10 days and 1 month using the modified Karlsson scoring method (maximum score 90)
    ≫ Pain (0 to 20)
    ≫ Swelling (0 to 10)
    ≫ Instability (subjective) (0 to 15)
    ≫ Stiffness (0 to 5)
    ≫ Stair climbing (0 to 10)
    ≫ Running (0 to 10)
    ≫ Work activities (0 to 15)
    ≫ Use of a support device (0 to 5)

- ▸ Secondary outcome measure
  - ▷ Difference in ankle girth at 10 days (circumferential measurement of the ankle at the level of both malleoli)
  - ▷ Difference in pain score at 10 days

Results

- ▸ Karlsson score
  - ▷ Significantly higher in the Aircast group at 10 days (*P* = 0.028)
    - » 50 in Aircast group
    - » 35 in elastic support bandage group
  - ▷ Significantly higher in the Aircast group at 1 month (*P* = 0.029)
    - » 68 in Aircast group
    - » 55 in elastic support bandage group
- ▸ No difference between the groups in the secondary outcome measures
  - ▷ Mean ankle girth
    - » Elastic bandage 14.4 mm
    - » Aircast ankle brace 8.5 mm (*P* = 0.09)
  - ▷ Mean pain score
    - » Elastic bandage 2.9
    - » Aircast 1.8 (*P* = 0.07)

Conclusion

- ▸ Use of an Aircast ankle brace for the treatment of lateral ligament ankle sprains produces a significant improvement in ankle joint function at both 10 days and 1 month compared with standard management with an elastic support bandage.

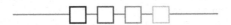

REVIEW ARTICLES

Anderson RB, Hunt KJ, McCormick JJ. Management of common sports-related injuries about the foot and ankle. *J Am Acad Orthop Surg.* 2010;18:546-556.

Nicola Maffulli N, Ferran NA. Management of acute and chronic ankle instability. *J Am Acad Orthop Surg.* 2008;16:608–615.

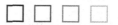

Achilles Tendon Injuries

Chapter **32**

FEATURED ARTICLE

Authors: Willits K, Amendola A, Bryant D, Mohtadi NG, Giffin JR, Fowler P, Kean CO, Kirkley A.

Title: Operative versus nonoperative treatment of acute Achilles tendon ruptures: a multicenter randomized trial using accelerated functional rehabilitation.

Journal Information: *J Bone Joint Surg.* 2010;92:2767–2775.

Study Design: Prospective Randomized Trial

- 145 patients with an acute Achilles tendon rupture randomized to:
  - Operative treatment (72 patients)
  - Nonoperative treatment (72 patients)
- Average age 40.4 years (22.5 to 67.2 years), 118 men, 26 women
- All patients underwent an accelerated rehabilitation protocol that featured early weight bearing and early range of motion.
- Outcome assessments
  - Primary outcome measurement at 3, 6, 12, and 24 months
    - » Rerupture rate as demonstrated by a positive Thompson squeeze test, presence of a palpable gap, and loss of plantar flexion strength
  - Secondary outcome measurement
    - » Isokinetic strength
    - » Leppilahti score

Miller MD, Mauffrey C, Hak DJ.
*Rapid Reference Review in Sports Medicine:
Pivotal Papers Revealed (pp 315-324).*
© 2016 Taylor & Francis Group.

> » Range of motion
> » Calf circumference

Results

- ▶ Rerupture
  - ▷ 2 patients in the operative group
  - ▷ 3 patients in the nonoperative group
- ▶ No clinically important difference between groups with regard to strength, range of motion, calf circumference, or Leppilahti
- ▶ Small but significant difference in plantar flexion strength ratio (affected to unaffected limb) at 240 degrees/s in favor of the operative treatment group
  - ▷ At 1 year mean difference 20.25% ($P = 0.05$)
  - ▷ At 2 years mean difference 14.15% ($P = 0.03$)
- ▶ Mean side-to-side difference in calf circumference (± standard deviation)
  - ▷ 1 year ($P = 0.99$)
    - » Operative group –1.3 cm (± 1.4 cm)
    - » Nonoperative group –1.3 cm (± 4.4 cm)
  - ▷ 2 years ($P = 0.75$)
    - » Operative group –1.7 cm (± 2.0 cm)
    - » Nonoperative group –1.5 cm (± 5.6 cm)
- ▶ Mean Leppilahti score (± standard deviation)
  - ▷ 1 year ($P = 0.53$)
    - » Operative group 78.5 (± 10.9)
    - » Nonoperative group 76.3 (± 15.8)
  - ▷ 2 years ($P = 0.89$)
    - » Operative group 82.6 (± 11.1)
    - » Nonoperative group 82.2 (± 12.3)
- ▶ Complications
  - ▷ 13 in the operative group
    - » 9 wound-healing complications, including 4 superficial infections and 1 deep infection
    - » 2 reruptures
    - » 1 deep vein thrombosis
    - » 1 pulmonary embolus
  - ▷ 6 in the nonoperative group
    - » 1 failure to heal with palpable gap
    - » 1 substantial pain
    - » 1 deep vein thrombosis
    - » 3 reruptures

Conclusions

▶ This study supports accelerated functional rehabilitation and nonoperative treatment for acute Achilles tendon ruptures (all but one prior study immobilized the limb for 6 to 8 weeks).

▶ All measured outcomes of nonoperative treatment were acceptable and were clinically similar to those for operative treatment.

▶ Treatment of Achilles tendon ruptures using a nonoperative protocol with accelerated rehabilitation avoids serious complications related to surgical management.

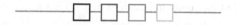

FEATURED ARTICLE

Author: Nistor L.

Title: Surgical and non-surgical treatment of Achilles tendon rupture. A prospective randomized study.

Journal Information: *J Bone Joint Surg Am.* 1981;63:394–399.

A Top 100 Cited Articles in Clinical Orthopedic Sports Medicine

---

Study Design: Prospective Randomized Trial

▶ 107 consecutive patients with acute Achilles tendon ruptures

▶ Treatment randomized based on day of presentation to hospital

  ▷ 2 were excluded (1 from each treatment group), leaving 105 patients

  ▷ Surgical (45 patients)

  ▷ Nonsurgical treatment (60 patients)

▶ Mean age 41 years (21 to 77 years), 96 men, 11 women

▶ Nonsurgical treatment protocol

  ▷ Immediate full weight bearing was permitted

  ▷ Below-the-knee plaster cast with ankle in gravity plantar flexion × 4 weeks

  ▷ Equinus angulation gently reduced and another cast applied

  ▷ Cast duration for most patients was 8 weeks (7 to 9 weeks)

  ▷ After final cast, a 2.5-cm heel lift added to shoes × 4 weeks or until able to dorsiflex 10 degrees

- ▶ Outcome assessments
  - ▷ Range of motion
  - ▷ Calf circumference
  - ▷ Tendon width
  - ▷ Plantar flexion strength
  - ▷ Ability to walk
  - ▷ Ability to stand on tiptoe
- ▶ Mean follow-up 2.5 years (1 to 5 years)

Results

- ▶ No significant difference in length of time off work
  - ▷ Surgical treatment group: average 13 weeks (0 to 30 weeks)
  - ▷ Nonoperative treatment group: average 9 weeks (0 to 44 weeks)
- ▶ Range of motion
  - ▷ Changes ≤5 degrees
    - » 27/41 surgically treated patients
    - » 40/54 nonoperatively treated patients
  - ▷ Changes ≥10 degrees
    - » 14/41 surgically treated patients
    - » 14/54 nonoperatively treated patients
- ▶ Achilles tendon width
  - ▷ Average increase 7 mm (2 to 12 mm) compared to contralateral side
  - ▷ Similar in both treatment groups
- ▶ Plantar flexion strength
  - ▷ No significant difference between the 2 treatment groups
- ▶ All patients could walk and stand on their tiptoes.
- ▶ Major complications
  - ▷ Surgical treatment group (45 patients)
    - ⟩ 2 reruptures
    - ⟩ 2 deep infections
  - » Nonoperative treatment group (60 patients)
    - ⟩ 5 reruptures
- ▶ Patient complaints (attributed to broadening of the Achilles tendon)
  - ▷ Difficulty with shoe wear
    - » 8 in surgical treatment group
    - » 1 in nonoperative treatment group
  - ▷ Ankle stiffness
    - » 22 in surgical treatment group
    - » 8 in nonoperative treatment group

Conclusions

▸ Author concluded that nonsurgical treatment offers advantages over surgical treatment.

▸ Only minor differences were noted between the final results in the 2 groups.

▸ Nonsurgical treatment had the advantages of shorter morbidity, fewer complaints, and no hospital stay.

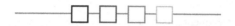

```
FEATURED ARTICLE

Authors: Twaddle BC, Poon P.

Title: Early motion for Achilles tendon ruptures: is surgery impor-
tant? A randomized, prospective study.

Journal Information: Am J Sports Med. 2007;35:2033–2038.
```

Study Design: Prospective Randomized Trial

▸ 42 patients with Achilles tendon rupture randomized to:
  ▷ Surgical treatment (20 patients)
  ▷ Nonoperative treatment (22 patients)

▸ Average age 41 years, 28 men, 14 women

▸ Both groups had early motion controlled in a removable orthosis and progressing to full weight bearing at 8 weeks from treatment.

▸ Inclusion criteria
  ▷ Presentation with 10 days of injury
  ▷ 18 to 50 years of age at time of injury
  ▷ Nonsmoker
  ▷ No other significant medical problems
  ▷ No medication use that may impair tendon healing

▸ Patients followed prospectively at 2, 8, 12, 26, or 52 weeks

▸ Outcome measurements
  ▷ Range of motion
  ▷ Calf circumference
  ▷ Musculoskeletal Functional Assessment Instrument (MFAI) outcome score

Results

- ▶ No significant differences between the 2 groups in MFAI scores, plantar flexion, dorsiflexion, or calf circumference
- ▶ Average MFAI outcome score at 52 weeks ($P = 0.64$)
  - ▷ Surgical treatment group 3.4
  - ▷ Nonoperative treatment group 4.2
- ▶ Average dorsiflexion difference (compared to contralateral ankle) at 52 weeks ($P = 0.061$)
  - ▷ Surgical treatment group –1
  - ▷ Nonoperative treatment group –0.2
- ▶ Average plantarflexion difference (compared to contralateral ankle) at 52 weeks ($P = 0.37$)
  - ▷ Surgical treatment group –0.6
  - ▷ Nonoperative treatment group –0.2
- ▶ Average calf circumference (compared to contralateral ankle) at 52 weeks ($P = 0.24$)
  - ▷ Surgical treatment group –0.5
  - ▷ Nonoperative treatment group –0.2
- ▶ Reruptures
  - ▷ 1 patient in each group was noncompliant and required surgical re-repair of a rerupture tendon after removing the orthosis and mobilizing without any splintage prior to 8 weeks.
  - ▷ 3 additional patients had a rerupture beyond the 8-week follow-up.
    - ≫ 2 in surgical treatment group
    - ≫ 1 in nonoperative treatment group
- ▶ No wound-healing complications in the operative treatment group

Conclusions

- ▶ Authors note that although several prior randomized studies have suggested improved outcome and superior strength with operative treatment, the nonoperatively treated patients in these studies have been immobilized for a much greater period of time and the surgically treated patients have been allowed controlled early motion and weight bearing.
- ▶ Early motion is an acceptable form of rehabilitation in both surgically and nonsurgically treated Achilles tendon ruptures.
- ▶ Authors concluded that surgical and nonoperative treatment produce comparable functional results and a low rerupture rate.

▶ Because there appears to be no difference between the 2 groups, the authors concluded that this suggests that controlled early motion is the important part of treatment of Achilles tendon ruptures.

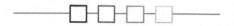

FEATURED ARTICLE

Authors: Soroceanu A, Sidhwa F, Aarabi S, Kaufman A, Glazebrook M.

Title: Surgical versus nonsurgical treatment of acute Achilles tendon rupture: a meta-analysis of randomized trials.

Journal Information: *J Bone Joint Surg Am.* 2012;94:2136–2143.

Study Design: Meta-analysis

▶ Examined published studies that compared surgical to nonoperative management of Achilles tendon ruptures.

▶ 10 randomized controlled studies met the inclusion criteria.

  ▷ 418 patients were treated surgically.

  ▷ 408 patients were treated nonoperatively.

  ▷ Patients were predominantly male.

  ▷ Mean patient age 39.8 years

Results

▶ Rerupture rates were equal for surgical and nonsurgical patients (risk difference = 1.7%, $P = 0.45$) when functional rehabilitation with early range of motion was used.

▶ If early range of motion was not used, the absolute risk reduction achieved by surgery was 8.8% ($P = 0.001$ in favor of surgery).

▶ Surgery was associated with an absolute risk increase of 15.8% ($P = 0.016$ in favor of nonoperative management) for complications other than rerupture.

▶ Surgical patients returned to work 19.16 days sooner ($P = 0.0014$).

▶ No significant difference between the 2 treatments with regard to:

  ▷ Calf circumference ($P = 0.357$)

  ▷ Strength ($P = 0.806$)

  ▷ Functional outcomes ($P = 0.226$)

Conclusions

▸ Conservative treatment should be considered at centers using functional rehabilitation.

▸ The use of functional rehabilitation resulted in rerupture rates similar to those for surgical treatment while offering the advantage of a decrease in other complications.

▸ Surgical repair should be preferred at centers that do not employ early range-of-motion protocols, as it decreased the rerupture risk in such patients.

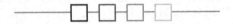

FEATURED ARTICLE

Authors: Metz R, Verleisdonk EJ, van der Heijden GJ, Clevers GJ, Hammacher ER, Verhofstad MH, van der Werken C.

Title: Acute Achilles tendon rupture: minimally invasive surgery versus nonoperative treatment with immediate full weightbearing. A randomized controlled trial.

Journal Information: *Am J Sports Med.* 2008;36:1688–1694.

Study Design: Prospective Randomized Trial

▸ 83 patients with acute Achilles tendon rupture randomized to:
  ▷ Nonoperative treatment of acute Achilles tendon rupture with functional bracing (41 patients)
  ▷ Minimally invasive surgical treatment followed by tape bandage (42 patients)
▸ All patients were allowed full weight bearing.
▸ Follow-up was 1 year
▸ 1 patient allocated to the surgical treatment group refused surgery and was treated nonoperatively.
▸ 2 patients allocated to the nonoperative treatment group refused and subsequently underwent surgery.
▸ Primary end point
  ▷ All complications other than reruptures

- ▶ Secondary end points
  - ▷ Time to return to work
  - ▷ Time to return to participation in sports
  - ▷ Patient satisfaction with treatment and pain measured on a 0 to 10 visual analog scale
- ▶ Follow-up visits at 1, 3, 5, and 7 weeks and at 3, 6, and 12 months
- ▶ Patient outcome at 6 months evaluated by the Leppilahti scoring method

Results

- ▶ Complications
  - ▷ No deep infections
  - ▷ 2 skin-related complications in the surgical treatment group
  - ▷ 13 skin-related complications in the nonoperative treatment group
  - ▷ Skin-related complications = fungal infection, pressure sores, blisters, and superficial wound infection
- ▶ Complications risk other than rerupture by intention-to-treat basis
  - ▷ 9/42 (21%) patients randomized to surgical treatment
  - ▷ 15/41 (36 %) patients randomized to nonoperative treatment
  - ▷ Risk ratio, 0.59; 95% confidence interval 0.29 to 1.19
- ▶ Rerupture
  - ▷ Intention-to-treat basis
    - » Rerupture in 5/41 patients randomized to nonoperative treatment
    - » Rerupture in 3/42 patients randomized to surgical treatment
    - » Risk ratio 0.59; 95% confidence interval 0.15 to 2.29
  - ▷ Actual treatment
    - » Rerupture in 6/40 (15%) patients following nonoperative treatment
    - » Rerupture in 2/43 (5%) patients following surgical treatment
    - » Risk ratio 0.31; 95% confidence interval 0.07 to 1.45; $P = 0.11$)
- ▶ Mean time to return to work
  - ▷ 59 days after surgical treatment
  - ▷ 108 days after nonoperative treatment
  - ▷ Difference = 49 days; 95% confidence interval 4 to 94; $P < 0.05$
- ▶ No significant difference in return to sports or treatment satisfaction
- ▶ Leppilahti score
  - ▷ No significant difference between treatment groups
  - ▷ 81% (26/32) good or excellent in surgical treatment group
  - ▷ 89% (24/27) good or excellent in nonoperative treatment group

Conclusions

▶ 15% lower risk of complications other than rerupture after minimally invasive surgical treatment and an absolute risk reduction of 41% favoring surgery, but these differences did not reach statistical significance.

▶ Authors concluded that there appeared to be a clinically important difference in the complication risk between minimally invasive surgical treatment and nonoperative treatment, but this difference did not reach statistical significance.

▶ Surgical treatment results in an earlier return to work.

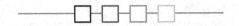

REVIEW ARTICLES

Chiodo CP, Glazebrook M, Bluman EM, et al. Diagnosis and treatment of acute Achilles tendon rupture *J Am Acad Orthop Surg.* 2010;18:503–513.

Saltzman CL, Tearse DS. Achilles tendon injuries. *J Am Acad Orthop Surg.* 1998;6:316–325.

Reddy SS, Pedowitz DI, Parekh SG, Omar IM, Wapner KL. Surgical treatment for chronic disease and disorders of the Achilles tendon. *J Am Acad Orthop Surg.* 2009;17:3–14.

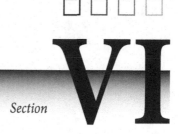

Section **VI**

Miscellaneous Topics

Concussion, Stress Fractures, Muscle Injury, Performance-Enhancing Drugs, and Sudden Cardiac Death

---

FEATURED ARTICLE: CONCUSSION

Authors: Guskiewicz KM, Weaver NL, Padua DA, Garrett WE Jr.

Title: Epidemiology of concussion in collegiate and high school football players.

Journal Information: *Am J Sports Med*. 2000;28:643–650.

A Top 100 Cited Articles in Clinical Orthopedic Sports Medicine

---

Study Design: Cohort Study

▸ Random sample survey of certified athletic trainers

▸ Survey population stratified by the athletic trainer employment setting (high school and collegiate divisions I, II, and III) and by the geographic district

▸ Athletic trainers instructed to complete a concussion report immediately after each concussion sustained by an athlete during the football season

▸ Received 242/392 surveys (62%) that were sent to high school and collegiate athletic trainers at the beginning of 3 football seasons (1995 to 1997)

▸ Authors investigated

  ▷ Incidence of injury

  ▷ Common signs and symptoms

  ▷ Patterns in making return-to-play decisions

Miller MD, Mauffrey C, Hak DJ.
*Rapid Reference Review in Sports Medicine:
Pivotal Papers Revealed (pp 327-332).*
© 2016 Taylor & Francis Group.

Results

- 5.1% (888/17,549) of football players sustained at least one concussion.
- Of these, 14.7% (131/888) sustained a second injury during the same season.
- Highest incidence of concussion was found at the high school (5.6%) and collegiate division III (5.5%) levels, which might be attributed to the increased exposure since these athletes often play both offense and defense at these levels.
- Players who sustained one concussion were 3 times more likely to sustain a second concussion in the same season than those players who did not sustain a prior injury.
- Severity of injury appeared to increase with recurrent injury.
  - ▷ Incidence of grade II concussion increased to 13% for those who reported one prior head injury in the past year.
  - ▷ Incidence of grade II concussion increased to 19% for those reporting more than one prior head injury.
- Contact with artificial turf appeared to be associated with a more serious concussion than contact with natural grass.
  - ▷ 22% of head contacts with artificial turf resulted in a grade II concussion.
  - ▷ 9% of head contacts with natural grass resulted in a grade II concussion.
- Common signs and symptoms
  - ▷ Only 8.9% of all injuries involved loss of consciousness.
  - ▷ 86% of all injuries involved a headache.
- Return-to-play decisions
  - ▷ 30.8% of all players sustaining a concussion returned to play on the same day of injury.
  - ▷ The remaining players returned to play at an average of only 4 days after a grade I concussion and after 8 days for a grade II concussion.
- Association between recurrent injury and the onset of selected symptoms
  - ▷ The total number of reported signs and symptoms associated with recurrent injury was 5.5, compared with only 3.5 for nonrecurrent injuries.
  - ▷ Amnesia
    - » Seen in 31% (78) of those players who had sustained a prior concussion within the last year
    - » Seen in 26% (189) of those players who had not sustained a prior concussion
  - ▷ Loss of consciousness
    - » 11% (28) in players who had sustained a prior concussion
    - » 8% in players who had not sustained a prior concussion

Conclusions

▸ Despite evolutionary changes in protective equipment, head injury remains common in football.

▸ High school and collegiate football players who sustain a concussion are nearly 3 times more likely to sustain a second concussion in the same season than those players who have not sustained a prior head injury.

▸ Clinicians do not follow the recommended guidelines for return to play, which call for:

   ▷ At least a 15- to 20-minute clearing period on the sideline

   ▷ Followed by a week of rest and monitoring of symptoms for those athletes who fail to clear quickly

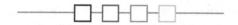

FEATURED ARTICLE: STRESS FRACTURES

Authors: Matheson GO, Clement DB, McKenzie DC, Taunton JE, Lloyd-Smith DR, Macintyre JG.

Title: Stress fractures in athletes. A study of 320 cases.

Journal Information: *Am J Sports Med.* 1987;15:46–58.

A Top 100 Cited Articles in Clinical Orthopedic Sports Medicine

---

Study Design: Retrospective Review

▸ Retrospective review and analysis of 320 athletes with bone scan–positive stress fractures (M = 145, F = 175) seen over 3.5 years

▸ Assessed the results of conservative management

▸ Mean age 26.7 years (13 to 61 years)

▸ Males were significantly older than females ($P = 0.0005$).

   ▷ Mean age for males 29.2 years

   ▷ Mean age for females 25.1 years

Results

▸ Localized tenderness and swelling are significant findings in stress fractures, but cannot be relied on as the sole criterion for the diagnosis.

- Distribution of stress fractures
  - ▷ 49.1% involved tibia
  - ▷ 25.3% involved tarsal bones
  - ▷ 8.8% involved metatarsals
  - ▷ 7.2% involved femur
  - ▷ 6.6% involved fibula
  - ▷ 1.6% involved pelvis
  - ▷ 0.9% involved sesamoid
  - ▷ 0.6% involved spine
- 16.6% of cases were bilateral.
- Significant difference in age among the sites
  - ▷ Femoral and tarsal stress fractures occurring in the oldest
  - ▷ Fibular and tibial stress fractures in the youngest
- Running was the most common sport at the time of injury, but there was no significant difference in weekly running mileage and affected sites.
- History of trauma was significantly more common for tarsal bone stress fractures.
- Average time to diagnosis 13.4 weeks (1 to 78 weeks)
- Average time to recovery 12.8 weeks (2 to 96 weeks)
- Time to diagnosis and recovery are site dependent.
  - ▷ Tarsal stress fractures took the longest time to diagnose and recover.
- Use of bone scans for diagnosis indicates that tarsal stress fractures are much more common than previously realized.

Conclusions

- Stress fractures should always be considered in the differential diagnosis of lower extremity pain in the athlete.
- Technetium[99] bone scan is the single most useful diagnostic aid.
- Patterns of stress fractures in athletes are different from those found in military recruits (who most frequently sustain stress fractures of the calcaneus or metatarsal).
- Conservative treatment of stress fractures in athletes is satisfactory in the majority of cases.
- The rehabilitation goal should be to return the athlete to full activity by reintroducing sport at a rate that allows remodeling adequate for the osseous system to meet the required physical stresses.

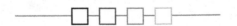

REVIEW ARTICLES: CONCUSSION

Durand P Jr, Adamson GJ. On-the-field management of athletic head injuries. *J Am Acad Orthop Surg.* 2004;12:191–195.

Uhl RL, Rosenbaum AJ, Cory Mulligan CM, King C. Minor traumatic brain injury: a primer for the orthopaedic surgeon. *J Am Acad Orthop Surg.* 2013;21:624–631.

REVIEW ARTICLES: MUSCLE INJURY

Beiner JM, Jokl P. Muscle contusion injuries: current treatment options. *J Am Acad Orthop Surg.* 2001;9:227–237.

Lieber RL, Friden J. Morphologic and mechanical basis of delayed-onset muscle soreness. *J Am Acad Orthop Surg.* 2002;10:67–73.

Maquirriain J, Merrelo M. The athlete with muscular cramps: clinical approach. *J Am Acad Orthop Surg.* 2007;15:425–431.

Noonan TJ, Garret WE Jr. Muscle strain injury: diagnosis and treatment. *J Am Acad Orthop Surg.* 1999;7:262–269.

REVIEW ARTICLES: PERFORMANCE-ENHANCING DRUGS

Silver MD. Use of ergogenic aids by athletes. *J Am Acad Orthop Surg.* 2001;9:61–70.

Yesalis CE, Bahrke MS. Anabolic-androgenic steroids and related substances. *Curr Sports Med Rep.* 2002,4:246–252.

REVIEW ARTICLES: STRESS FRACTURES

Boden BP, Osbahr DC. High-risk stress fractures: evaluation and treatment. *J Am Acad Orthop Surg.* 2000;8:344–353.

Shindle MK, Endo Y, Warren RF, et al. Stress fractures about the tibia, foot, and ankle. *J Am Acad Orthop Surg.* 2012;20:167–176.

REVIEW ARTICLES: SUDDEN CARDIAC DEATH

Maron BJ. Sudden death in young athletes. *N Engl J Med*. 2003;349:1064–1075.

Maron BJ, Thompson PD, Ackerman MJ, et al. Recommendations and considerations related to preparticipation screening for cardiovascular abnormalities in competitive athletes: 2007 update. A scientific statement from the American Heart Association council on nutrition, physical activity, and metabolism. Endorsed by the American College of Cardiology Foundation. *Circulation*. 2007;115:1643–1655.

Financial Disclosures

Dr. Megan M. Gleason has no financial or proprietary interest in the materials presented herein.

Dr. David J. Hak has no financial or proprietary interest in the materials presented herein.

Dr. Cyril Mauffrey has no financial or proprietary interest in the materials presented herein.

Dr. Mark D. Miller is the founder and director of the Miller Review Course and receives royalties from Elsevier and Wolters-Kluwer.

Dr. Jeff Tuman has no financial or proprietary interest in the materials presented herein.

Printed in the United States
by Baker & Taylor Publisher Services